The American Civil War Medical Series

Ira M. Rutkow, M.D., Dr.P.H.

1. John Ordronaux. *Hints on the Preservation of Health in Armies*. New York: 1861. BOUND WITH: Ordronaux. *Manual of Instructions for Military Surgeons*. New York: 1863.
2. Joseph Janvier Woodward. *The Hospital Steward's Manual*. Philadelphia: 1862.
3. Frank Hastings Hamilton. *A Practical Treatise on Fractures and Dislocations*. Philadelphia: 1860.
4. Francis Peyre Porcher. *Resources of the Southern Fields and Forests, Medical, Economical, and Agricultural*. Richmond: 1863.
5. William Alexander Hammond. *A Treatise on Hygiene*. Philadelphia: 1863.
6. Roberts Bartholow. *A Manual of Instructions for Enlisting and Discharging Soldiers*. Philadelphia: 1863.
7. Claude Bernard and Charles Huette. *Illustrated Manual of Operative Surgery and Surgical Anatomy*. Edited, with notes and additions . . . by William H. Van Buren and Charles E. Isaacs. New York: 1861.
8. Samuel Preston Moore. *Regulations of the C.S.A. Medical Department* IN: *Regulations for the Army of the Confederate States*. Richmond: 1862.
9. Charles Ravenscroft Greenleaf. *A Manual for the Medical Officers of the United States Army*. Philadelphia: 1864.
10. William Grace. *The Army Surgeon's Manual*. New York: 1864.
11. Joseph Janvier Woodward. *Outlines of the Chief Camp Diseases of the United States Armies*. Philadelphia: 1863.
12. *Confederate States Medical and Surgical Journal*. Richmond: January 1864 – February 1865.

THE ARMY SURGEON'S MANUAL

THE ARMY SURGEON'S MANUAL

For the Use of Medical Officers, Cadets, Chaplains, and Hospital Stewards

by William Grace

Reprinted with a Biographical Introduction by Ira M. Rutkow, M.D., Dr.P.H.

Norman Publishing
San Francisco
1992

Published by Norman Publishing
720 Market Street
San Francisco, California 94102–2502

Library of Congress Cataloging-in-Publication Data

Grace, William.
The army surgeon's manual / by William Grace ; reprinted with a biographical introduction by Ira M. Rutkow.
p. cm. — (The American Civil War medical series ; 10)
Reprint. Originally published: New York : Bailliere Brothers, 1864.
Includes index.
ISBN 0–930405–41–2 (alk. paper)
1. Surgery, Operative. 2. Medicine, Military. I. Rutkow, Ira. II. Title. III. Series.
[DNLM: 1. Military Medicine. 2. Surgery, Operative. UH G729a 1864a]
RD151.G69 1991
616.93′8023—dc20
DNLM/DLC
for Library of Congress 90–14278
CIP

The American Civil War Medical Series, No. 10

This book was reproduced from the original edition loaned from the Francis A. Countway Library of Medicine, Boston.

This book is printed on acid-free paper, and its binding materials have been chosen for strength and durability.

Manufactured in the United States of America.

WILLIAM GRACE

There is little biographical information available about William Grace. What is known was obtained from the pension records of Civil War army officers, which are now held in the National Archives in Washington, D.C. (among them personal papers of surgeons and *Records of the Office of the Adjutant General* [Office Record Group 94]). Grace first served in the U.S. Army when he was drafted and appointed as a hospital steward on May 20, 1857. He was initially assigned to duty in Texas, and although he was most likely stationed at other posts during his tour of duty, this remains conjecture. Regardless, he was honorably discharged on December 12, 1860, for "reason of expiration of term of service." It is believed that

Grace was from the District of Columbia because it was from that area that he was first drafted. Since the average age of the pre-Civil War draftee was in the early twenties, it can be reasonably assumed that Grace was born sometime in the 1830s.

The status of the army's hospital stewards prior to the Civil War was often muddled. The level of aid that properly trained stewards supplied for surgeons ranged from simple administrative tasks to apothecary's duties and even the performance of minor surgical operations. The demand for their services was great and since the army's medical department was chronically shortstaffed of physicians, a competent hospital steward was an invaluable assistant. In 1856 Congress granted the secretary of war the authority to begin hiring more civilians to be permanently attached to the medical department as hospital stewards for a salary of thirty dollars a month. This law also granted men who served as cooks and nurses extra duty pay in recognition of the hazardous and unpleasant nature of much of their work. Unfortunately, the attempt to create an efficient and self-contained corps of stewards was never completed, and by 1861 they still remained in short supply.

With the beginning of the Civil War, Grace decided to re-enlist and did so on June 3, 1861, this time from New York. He was immediately assigned to clerical duty in the surgeon general's office in Washington with his old rank of hospital steward. Grace remained there until December 8, 1862, when he was again discharged with the intent of being immediately employed as an acting assistant surgeon on duty in the surgeon general's office.

The acting assistant surgeons were also known as the "contract" surgeons. They held no commission but received the pay of first lieutenants. There were over 5,500 such individuals and most served for only three to six months. Candidates were expected to be medical school graduates and were supposed to pass examinations before boards established by the U.S. Army Medical Department. Yet, it was often charged that unfit persons were employed: some had never seen the inside of a professional school. Through 1864 pay for full time service was from eighty to one hundred dollars a month and it might not be unreasonable to assume that this salary was why Grace wanted to work as an acting assistant surgeon.

When and where Grace received his medical education is uncertain. Whether he even received a M.D. is unknown because on the title page of the *Army Surgeon's Manual* he is listed only as "William Grace of Washington, D.C." Perhaps Grace received the title and pay of a medical officer without ever receiving a formal medical education because of his previous service in the surgeon general's office. It is not even apparent that Grace was in the army when he helped edit this work or why he gave up his status as an acting assistant surgeon prior to the conclusion of the war. *The Army Surgeon's Manual* was first published in the fall of 1864. It contained regulations of the medical department, all general orders from the war department, and circulars from the surgeon general's office from January 1, 1861, to July 1, 1864. A second, somewhat larger, edition was issued in 1865. These two editions remain the only complete source for the rules and regulations of the army's medical department. As far as can be determined, the *Manual* is the only written work that Grace ever produced.

Grace died from unstated causes on November 5, 1865. He is known to have been married because in 1879 his widow began a series of claims for pension benefits secondary to his military service. No disability is noted in his records and whether any benefits were paid is uncertain. It remains undetermined as to whether Grace had any children.

THE

ARMY SURGEON'S MANUAL,

FOR THE USE OF

MEDICAL OFFICERS, CADETS, CHAPLAINS, AND HOSPITAL STEWARDS,

CONTAINING THE

REGULATIONS OF THE MEDICAL DEPARTMENT, ALL GENERAL ORDERS FROM THE WAR DEPARTMENT, AND CIRCULARS FROM THE SURGEON-GENERAL'S OFFICE.

From January 1st, 1861, to July 1st, 1864.

BY WILLIAM GRACE,

OF WASHINGTON, D.C.

Published by permission of the Surgeon-General.

NEW YORK:

BAILLIERE BROTHERS, 520 BROADWAY.

1864.

R. CRAIGHEAD,
Printer, Stereotyper, and Electrotyper,
Carton Building,
81, 83, *and* 85 *Centre Street.*

CONTENTS.

ARMY SURGEON'S MANUAL.

PART I.

LIST OF THE MEDICAL STAFF, U. S. ARMY, JULY 1, 1864.

REGULARS.

SURGEON-GENERAL

(RANKING AS BRIGADIER-GENERAL),

William A. Hammond.*

ASSIST. SURG.-GENERAL

(RANKING AS COLONEL),

Robert C. Wood.

MEDICAL INSPECTOR-GENERAL

(RANKING AS COLONEL),

Joseph K. Barnes.†

MEDICAL INSPECTORS

(RANKING AS LIEUT.-COLONEL).

John M. Cuyler,
Richard H. Coolidge,
Charles C. Keeney,
Edward P. Vollum,
George H. Lyman,
George T. Allen,
Lewis Humphreys,
Peter Pineo,
Augustus C. Hamlin,
George K. Johnson,
John E. Summers.
N. S. Townsend,
George W. Stipp,
John Wilson,
John L. Le Conte,
E. D. Kittoe.

---

* Surgeon-General Hammond, dismissed August 20, 1864.

† Medical Inspector-General Barnes, appointed Surgeon-General, August 22, 1864.

SURGEONS

(RANKING AS MAJOR).

Richard S. Satterlee,
Charles S. Tripler,
Charles McDougall,
Burton Randall,
Adam N. McLaren,
Joseph J. B. Wright,
Madison Mills,
Eugene H. Abadie,
Charles McCormick,
Charles H. Laub,
Josiah Simpson,
William J. Sloan,
William S. King,
James Simons,
Levi H. Holden,
Robert Murray,
John F. Head,
Lewis A. Edwards,
John F. Hammond,
Elisha J. Baily,
George E. Cooper,
Ebenezer Swift,
Glover Perin,
Peter G. S. Ten Broeck,
John Campbell,
Charles H. Crane,
Thomas A. McParlin,
Joseph B. Brown,
Alexander B. Hasson,
Jonathan Letterman,
Robert O. Abbott,
Thomas L Getty,
David L. Magruder,
John J. Milhau,
Horace R. Wirtz,
Charles Page,
Charles Sutherland,
Basil Norris,
John Moore,
Andrew K. Smith,
Richard H. Alexander,
Joseph R. Smith,
James T. Ghiselin,
John F. Randolph,
George Taylor,
Bernard J. D. Irwin,
Anthony Heger,
Charles J. Alexander,
Bennett A. Clements,
Lewis Taylor.

ASSISTANT-SURGEONS

(RANKING AS CAPTAIN).

Joseph C. Baily
J. Cooper McKee.

(RANKING AS FIRST LIEUTENANT).

Joseph H. Bill,
De Witt C. Peters,
Charles H. Alden,
Warren Webster,
John Vansant,
Charles C. Byrne,
J. Campbell Shorb,
Abel F. Mechem,
Clinton Wagner,
William F. Cornick,
Joseph P. Wright,
Havilah M. Sprague,
Charles C. Gray,
William C. Spencer,
Francis L. Town,
Alexander Ingram,
Peter V. Schenck,
Dallas Bache,
Blencowe E. Fryer,
John H. Frantz,
Walter Lindsly,
Charles E. Goddard,

Henry R. Silliman,
Philip C. Davis,
Joseph S. Smith,
Charles I. Wilson,
James F. Weeds,
Charles B. White,
George M. Sternberg,
Laurence H. Sheldon,
Joseph J. Woodward,
Edward S. Dunster,
Elias J. Marsh,
Robert F. Weir,
Thomas C. Brainerd,
Morris J. Asch,
Henry S. Schell,
Charles K. Winne,
Joseph H. Semple,
William H. Forwood,
Ely McClellan,
Charles A. McCall,
Samuel A. Storrow,
John C. C. Downing,
William D. Wolverton,
William R. Ramsey,
Thomas H. Helsby,
Albert Hartsuff,
Charles R. Greenleaf,
Philip Adolphus,
Bolivar Knickerbocker,
John V. D. Middleton,
William Thomson,
John Bell,
John H. Janeway,
Henry A. DuBois,
Benjamin Howard,
Henry C. Parry,
Henry R. Tilton,
Samuel M. Horton,
John C. G. Happersett,
Alfred A. Woodhull,
William A. Bradley,
George P. Jaquett,
William T. Okie,
John S. Billings,
Samuel Adams,
Phineas S. Conner,
Thomas G. MacKenzie,
William M. Notson,
E. de W. Breneman,
George M. McGill,
Jeremiah B. Brinton,
William E. Waters,
Joseph R. Gibson,
Cyrus Bacon,
Samuel H. Horner,
George L. Porter,
David L. Huntington,
John W. Williams,
Charles M. Colton,
Justus M. Brown,
Charles S. De Graw,
Edward C. Strode,
Andrew H. Smith,
Van Buren Hubbard,
Harrison Allen,
William P. Grier,
Thomas McMillin,
Edward Brooks,
Thomas H. Ridgely,
Charles C. Lee,
Samuel H. Orton,
John W. Brewer,
John Homans,
John Brooke,
William F. Gardner,
Harvey E. Brown,
J. Theodore Calhoun,
Edward J. Darken,
William E. Whitehead,
William F. Norris,
Edward Cowles,
Michael Hillary,
Edward Curtis,
Charles Smart,
Elliott Coues,
William F. Buchanan,
J. H. Kinsman.

VOLUNTEERS.

SURGEONS

(RANKING AS MAJOR).

Henry S. Hewitt,
John H. Brinton,
John A. Lidell,
George Suckley,
Samuel W. Gross,
Alex. H. Hoff,
Rufus H. Gilbert,
Charles McMillan,
Charles O'Leary,
A. B. Campbell,
James V. Z. Blaney,
John S. Bobbs,
John H. Rauch,
William D. Stewart,
Nathaniel R. Derby,
A. E. Stocker,
Joshua Owen,
Thomas Rush Spencer,
William Clendenin,
George G. Shumard,
William Varian,
Orlando M. Bryan,
Thomas H. Bache,
James D. Strawbridge,
Josiah Curtis,
Francis Noel Burke,
R. B. McCay,
John J. Craven,
Robert L. Stanford,
Edwin Bentley,
Reed B. Bontecou,
D. W. Bliss,
H. P. Stearns,
George H. Oliver,.
Alex. N. Dougherty,
George H. Hubbard,
D. W. Hand,
Thomas Antisell,
John McNulty,
Daniel Meeker,
Gideon S. Palmer,
John H. Taylor,
William M. Chambers,
J. H. Grove,
A. Henry Thurston,
Oliver A. Judson,
T. F. Azpell,
Christ. C. Cox,
Gabriel Grant,
John G. Keenan,
Charles W. Jones,
George L. Pancoast,
Nathaniel R. Mosely,
F. H. Gross,
David J. McKibbin,
Robert Niccolls,
Thomas Sim,
George S. Kemble,
Thomas F. Perley,
Milton Goldsmith,
James Bryan,
Robert A. Christian,
A. R. Egbert,
C. F. H. Campbell,
William Hayes,
Eugene F. Sanger,
Robert K. Smith,
David P. Smith,
J. B. G. Baxter,
Lavington Quick,
Norman Gay,
George Rex,
Thomas A. Worrall,
Meredith Clymer,
Thomas W. Fry,
Edward E. Phelps,
Alex. T. Watson,
J. H. Boucher,
J. H. Baxter,
William H. Thorn,
Jacob Bockee,
Abraham Crispell,
Thomas B. Reed,
Horace Wardner,
J. B. Lewis,
James C. Fisher,

James G. Hatchitt,
Abram L. Cox,
Alonzo J. Phelps,
William Dickinson,
Ira Russell,
Isaac I. Hayes,
Henry Palmer,
Clark McDermont,
George M. Kellogg,
Artemas Chapel,
John T. Heard,
A. P. Dalrymple,
Burkitt Cloak,
Adam Hammer,
Edward McDonnell,
Charles L. Allen,
Henry Buckmaster,
Morse K. Taylor,
Francis Bacon,
John Neil,
Alfred Wynkoop,
Thomas R. Crosby,
Edward Shippen,
Zenas E. Bliss,
Henry J. Churchman,
Paul B. Goddard,
Joseph Hopkinson,
Henry A. Martin,
John R. McClurg,
Clayton A. Cowgill,
Bowman B. Breed,
Silvanus D. Freeman,
Israel Moses,
James C. Whitehill,
Alexander B. Mott,
Pliny A. Jewett,
John O. Bronson.
David Stanton,
F. S. Ainsworth,
Francis Salter,
Howard Culbertson,
Augustus M. Clark,
Sylvanus S. Mulford,
Daniel G. Brinton,
John E. Herbst,
Joseph S. Hildreth,
John H. Phillips,
James M. McNulty,
R. M. S. Jackson,
Socrates N. Sherman,
John M. Robinson,
Samuel B. Davis,
E. W. Thurm,
Jacob R. Ludlow,
J. D. Brumley,
Ferdinand V. Hayden,
Sanford B. Hunt,
William H. Gobrecht,
George R. Weeks,
Benjamin B. Wilson,
Henry Janes,
B. A. Vanderkieft,
Edward B. Dalton,
William S. Thomson.
Samuel D. Turney,
John W. Foye,
George L. Sutton,
Alfred F. Sheldon,
Peter Cleary,
Robert R. Taylor,
Caleb W. Horner,
Edward J. Whitney,
Seymour D. Carpenter,
R. S. Kenderdine,
John E. McDonald,
Cyrus N. Chamberlain,
William A. Conover,
Frederick A. Keffer,
Lewis D. Harlow,
Elmore Y. Chase,
Conrad C. Dumreecher,
Henry A. Schlaefflin,
J. W. Pittinos,
John Bradley,
A. M. Speer,
Robert Reyburn,
S. E. Fuller,
G. F French,
P. A. O'Connell,
J. William Lawton,
St. John W. Mintzer,
J. B. Morrison,
A. M. Wilder,
Philip Harvey,
James B. Bellangee,
John L. Teed,
Louis W. Reed,
J. J. De Lamater,

A. C. Schwarzwelder,
William Threlkeld,
Frank Meacham,
Charles E. Swasey,
J. H. Bayne,
George W. Hogeboom,
Lewis C. Rice,
James H. Peabody,
William R. Dewitt,
Henry W. Ducachet,
William Watson,
Richard D. Lynde,
William Grinsted,
J. H. Currey,
Nathan P. Rice,
S. Atherton Holman,
Charles S. Wood,
Samuel Kneeland,
M. K. Hogan,
Abel C. Benedict,
John Trenor,
Jabez Perkins,
Francis Greene,
Frederick Lloyd,
Robert Fletcher,
A. C. Van Duyn,
Lincoln R. Stone,
William C. Bennett,
Edward P. Morong,
Otis M. Humphrey,
J. H. Thompson,
Roger W. Pease,
Charles S. Frink,
George A. Wheeler,
James M. Laing,
Samuel Hart,
Charles J. Kipp,
S. S. Schultz,
J. K. Rogers,
N. S. Barnes,
James M. Leete,
N. F. Marsh,
Henry Eversman,
Charles B. White,
Joel Seaverns,
J. Y. Cantwell,
William I. Wolfley,
H. Earnest Goodman,
Henry L. W. Burritt,
Isaac D. Knight,
Edward A. Clark,
Thomas B. Hood,
George Derby,
H. Z. Gill,
John C. Norton,
W. C. Daniels.

ASSISTANT-SURGEONS

(RANKING AS FIRST LIEUTENANT).

A. B. Chapin,
J. W. Applegate,
John D. Johnson,
Hor. B. Buck,
Dennis B. Hannan,
J. W. Merriam,
Harley P. Mathewson,
M. King Moxley,
William W. Wythes,
Charles F. Haynes,
John Q. Adams,
Franklin Grube,
Henry T. Legler
William Carroll,
Walter O. McDonald,
William A. Banks,
Washington B. Trull,
George McC. Miller,
Frank Reynolds,
John H. Doughty,
J. A. White,
George S. Courtright,
William S. Ely,
Henry C. Roberts,
Calvin C. Chaffee,
Robert McGowan,
Rudolf Tauszky,
George S. Rose,
G. A. Mursick,
J. M. Study,

Charles F. Brisbane,
E. D. Buckman,
A. M. Sigmund,
John F. Huber,
Henry M. Kirke,
C. H. Hood,
J. A. Freeman,
Theodore Artaud,
John C. Carter,
J. McCurdy,
M. C. Woodworth,
Samuel Kitchen,
Frederick Wolf,
A. E. Carothers,
A. P. Williams,
Alfred Delany,
W. S. Woods,
J. S. Radcliffe,
L. D. Sheets,
Benjamin McCluer,
Aug. Van Cleef,
John Collins,
A. I. Comfort,
Theodore A. McGraw,
S. B. Ward,
J. Sykes Ely,
Herman Loewenthal,
N. M. Glatfelter,
Gerhard Saal,
Patrick Glennan,
Edward M. Powers,
Brinton Stone,
Benjamin Durham,
A. McMahon,
J. B. Petherbridge,
M. B. Cochran,
H. W. Davis,
Daniel R. Brower,
Thomas R. Pooley,
J. H. Ledlie,
Mason F. Cogswell,
George P. De Grassi,
Nelson S. Drake,
W. S. Millener,
E. Griswold,
W. A. Harvey,
H. G. Keefer,
Thomas H. Sherwood,
Thomas G. Henry,
George A. Otis,
Ebenezer McClintock,
J. B. Cutts,
E. W. Mills.

MEDICAL STOREKEEPERS.

Hennel Stevens,
Henry M. Rittenhouse,
Henry Johnson,
Robert T. Creamer,
George Wright.

PART II.

REGULATIONS OF THE MEDICAL DEPARTMENT, FROM THE REVISED REGULATIONS FOR THE ARMY.

(Approved August 10, 1861.)

ARTICLE XLIV.

MEDICAL DEPARTMENT.

1266. The medical supplies for the army are prescribed in the standard supply tables.

1267. The medical purveyors and the senior medical officer of each hospital, post, or command, will make the necessary requisitions for medical and hospital supplies, in duplicate (Form 1). If the supplies are to be obtained from the principal purveying depôts, the requisitions will be made upon the Surgeon-General on the 31st day of December annually; if from department or field depôts, they will be made upon the medical director at such times and for such periods as he may direct. Good vaccine matter will be kept on hand by timely requisition on the Surgeon-General.

1268. The medical purveyors at the principal depôts will issue medical and hospital supplies only on the order of the Surgeon-General; those at department or field depôts will issue on the order of a medical director. In particular and urgent cases, issues may be made on a special requisition (Form 2), approved by a commanding officer; a like authority will be required in transfers of medical supplies.

1269. When it is necessary to purchase medical supplies, and recourse cannot be had to a medical disbursing officer, they may be procured by the quartermaster on a special requisition (Form 2) and account (Form 3).

1270. When any requisition for medical supplies is not according to the supply table, the reason therefor must be set out.

1271. In every case of special requisition, a duplicate of the requisition shall, at the same time, be transmitted to the Surgeon-General for his information, giving the name and station of the officer upon whom it is made.

1272. Medical purveyors will make to the Surgeon-General, at the end of each fiscal quarter, returns in duplicate (Form 4) of medical supplies received, issued, and remaining on hand, stating to whom, or from whom, and where and when issued or received; other medical officers in charge of medical supplies make similar returns of them annually, on the 31st December; and all officers, when relieved from the duty to which their returns relate. The returns will show the condition of the stores, and particularly of the instruments, bedding, and furniture. Medical purveyors will furnish abstracts of receipts and issues, with their returns (Form 5), giving the name of the person from whom received and to whom issued.

1273. An officer transferring medical supplies will furnish a certified invoice to the officer who is to receive them, and transmit a duplicate of it to the Surgeon-General. The receiving officer will furnish a receipt to the officer making the issue, with a report of the quality and condition of the articles, and transmit a duplicate of the receipt and report to the Surgeon-General. A medical officer who turns over medical supplies to a quartermaster for storage or transportation will forward to the Surgeon-General, with the invoice, the quartermaster's receipt for the packages.

1274. Medical officers will take up and account for all medical supplies of the army that come into their possession, and report, when they know it, to whose account they are to be credited.

1275. In all official lists of medical supplies the articles will be entered in the order of the supply table.

1276. Medical disbursing officers will, at the end of each fiscal quarter, render to the Surgeon-General, in duplicate, a quarterly account current of moneys received and expended, with the proper vouchers for the payments, and certificates that the services have been rendered, and the supplies purchased and received for the medical service, and transmit to him an estimate of the funds required for the next quarter.

1277. The senior medical officer of a hospital will distribute the patients, according to convenience and the nature of their complaints, into wards or divisions, under the particular charge of the several assistant-surgeons, and will visit them himself each day, as frequently as the state of the sick may require, accompanied by the assistant, steward, and nurse.

1278. His prescriptions of medicine and diet are written down at once in the proper register, with the name of the patient and the number of his bed; the assistants fill up the diet table for the day, and direct the administration of the prescribed medicines. He will detail an assistant-surgeon to remain at the hospital day and night, when the state of the sick requires it.

1279. In distributing the duties of his assistants, he will ordinarily require the aid of one in the care and preparation of the hospital reports, registers, and records, the rolls and descriptive lists; and of another in the charge of the dispensary, instruments, medicines, hospital expenditures, and the preparation of the requisitions and annual returns.

1280. He will enforce the proper hospital regulations to promote health and prevent contagion, by ventilated and not crowded rooms, scrupulous cleanliness, frequent changes of bedding, linen, &c.

1281. He will require the steward to take due care of the hospital stores and supplies; to enter in a book, daily (Form 6), the issues to the ward-masters, cooks, and nurses; to prepare the provision returns, and receive and distribute the rations.

1282. He will require the ward-master to take charge of the effects of the patients; to register them in a book (Form 7); to have them numbered and labelled with the patient's name, rank, and company; to receive from the steward the furniture, bedding, cooking-utensils, etc., for use, and keep a record of them (Form 8), and how distributed to the wards and kitchens; and once a week to take an inventory of the articles in use, and report to him any loss or damage to them, and to return to the steward such as are not required for use.

1283. The cooks and nurses are under the orders of the steward; he is responsible for the cleanliness of the wards and kitchens, patients and attendants, and all articles in use. He will ascertain who are present at sunrise, and sunset, and tattoo, and report absentees.

1284. At surgeon's call the sick then in the companies will be conducted to the hospital by the first sergeants, who will each hand to the surgeon, in his company-book, a list of all the sick of the company, on which the surgeon shall state who are to remain or go into hospital; who are to return to quarters as sick or convalescent; what duties the convalescents in quarters are capable of; what cases are feigned; and any other information in regard to the sick of the company he may have to communicate to the company commander.

1285. Soldiers in hospital, patients, or attendants, except stewards, shall be mustered on the rolls of their company, if it be present at the post.

1286. When a soldier in hospital is detached from his company so as not to be mustered with it for pay, his company commander shall certify and send to the hospital his descriptive list, and account of pay and clothing, containing all necessary information relating to his accounts with the United States, on which the surgeon shall enter all payments, stoppages, and issues of clothing to him in hospital. When he leaves the hospital, the medical officer shall certify and remit his descriptive list, showing the state of his accounts. If he is discharged from the service in hospital, the surgeon shall make out his final statements for pay and clothing. If he dies in hospital, the surgeon shall take charge of his effects, and make the reports required in the general regulations concerning soldiers who die absent from their companies.

1287. Patients in hospital are, if possible, to leave their arms and accoutrements with their companies, and in no case to take ammunition into the hospital.

1288. When a patient is transferred from one hospital to another, the medical officer shall send with him an account of his case, and the treatment.

1289. The regulations for the service of hospitals apply, as far as practicable, to the medical service in the field.

1290. The senior medical officer of each hospital, post, regiment, or detachment, will keep the following records, and deliver them to his successor; a register of patients (Form 9); a prescription book (Form 10); a diet book (Form 10); a case book; a meteorological register (Form 11); copies of his requisitions, annual returns, and quarterly reports of sick and wounded; and an order and letter-book, in which will be transcribed all orders and letters relating to his duties.

1291. He will make up the muster and pay rolls of the medical cadets, hospital steward, female nurses, and matrons, and of all soldiers in hospital, sick or on duty, detached from their companies, on the forms furnished from the Adjutant-General's office, and according to the directions expressed on them.

1292. He will make the rolls of the cooks and nurses for extra-duty pay, which will be paid by the paymaster, in the absence of a medical disbursing officer, as in other cases of expenditures for the medical department (Form 12).

1293. The senior medical officer will select the cooks, nurses, and matrons (and, at posts where there is no hospital steward appointed by the Secretary of War, a soldier to act as steward), with the approval of the commanding officer. Cooks and nurses will be taken from the privates, and will be exempt from other duty, but shall attend the parades for muster and weekly inspections of their companies at the post, unless specially excused by the commanding officer.

1294. Ordinarily, hospital attendants are allowed as follows: to a General Hospital, one steward, one nurse as ward-master, one nurse to ten patients, one matron to twenty, and one cook to thirty; to a hospital where the command exceeds five companies, one steward and ward-master, one cook, two matrons, and four nurses; to a post or garrison of one company, one steward and ward-master, one nurse, one cook, and one matron; and for every two companies more, one nurse; at arsenals where the number of enlisted men is not less than fourteen, one matron is allowed. The allowance of hospital attendants for troops in the field will be, for one company, one steward, one nurse, and one cook; for each additional company, one nurse; and for commands of over five companies, one additional cook.

1295. Medical officers, where on duty, will attend the officers and enlisted men, and the servants and laundresses authorized by law; and at stations where other medical attendance cannot be procured, and on marches, the hired men of the army, and the families of officers and soldiers. Medicines will be dispensed to the families of officers and soldiers, and to all persons entitled to medical attendance; hospital stores to enlisted men.

1296. Medical officers, in giving certificates of disability (Form 13), are to take particular care in all cases that have not been under their charge; and especially in epilepsy, convulsions, chronic rheumatism, derangement of the urinary organs, ophthalmia, ulcers, or any obscure disease liable to be feigned or purposely produced; and in no case shall such certificate be given until after sufficient time and examination to detect any attempt at deception.

1297. In passing a recruit the medical officer is to examine him stripped; to see that he has free use of all his limbs; that his chest is ample; that his hearing, vision, and speech are perfect; that he has no tumors, or ulcerated or extensively cicatrised legs; no rupture or chronic cutaneous affection; that he has not received any contusion, or wound of the head, that may impair his faculties; that he is not a drunkard; is not subject to convulsions; and has no infectious disorder, nor any other that may unfit him for military service.

1298. Medical officers attending recruiting rendezvous will keep a record (Form 14) of all the recruits examined by them. Books for this purpose will be procured by application to the Surgeon-General, to whom they will be returned when filled.

1299. As soon as a recruit joins any regiment or station, he shall be examined by the medical officer, and vaccinated when it is required.

1300. The senior medical officer of each hospital, post, regiment, or detachment, will make monthly to the medical director, and quarterly to the Surgeon-General, a report of sick and wounded, and of deaths, and of certificates for discharge for disability (Form 15), and transmit to him monthly a copy of the meteorological register (Form 11), and a copy of the "statement of the hospital fund" (Form 19).

1301. After surgeon's call, he will make a morning report of the sick to the commanding officer (Form 16).

1302. Every medical officer will report to the Surgeon-General and to the medical director the date when he arrives at a station, or when he leaves it, and his orders in the case, and at the end of each month whenever not at his station, whether on service or on leave of absence, and when on leave of absence his post-office address for the next month.

1303. The medical director will make to the Surgeon-General a monthly return of the medical officers of the command (Form 17), and a consolidated monthly report of the sick and wounded (Form 15) from the several reports made to him.

1304. When it is necessary to employ a private physician as medical officer, the commanding officer may do it by written contract, conditioned as in Form 18, at a stated compensation not to exceed $50 a month when the number of officers and men, with authorized servants and laundresses, is 100 or more; $40 when it is from 50 to 100, and $30 when it is under 50.

1305. But when he is required to abandon his own business, and give his whole time to the public service, the contract may be not to exceed $80 a month; and not to exceed $100, besides transportation in kind, to be furnished by the Quartermaster's Department, where he is required to accompany troops on marches or transports. But a private physician will not be employed to accompany troops on marches or transports, except by orders from the War Department, or in particular and urgent cases by the order of the officer directing the movement, when a particular statement of the circumstances which make it necessary will be appended to the contract.

1306. And when a private physician is required to furnish medicines, he will be allowed, besides the stipulated pay, from 25 to 50 per cent. on it, to be determined by the Surgeon-General.

1307. In all cases, a duplicate of the contract will be transmitted forthwith by the commanding officer to the Surgeon-General, and the commanding officer for the time being will at once discontinue it, whenever the necessity for it ceases, or the Surgeon-General may so direct.

1308. The physician's account of pay due must be sent to the Surgeon-General for payment, vouched by the certificate of the commanding officer that it is correct and agreeable to contract, and that the services have been duly rendered. But when it cannot conveniently be submitted to the Surgeon-General from the frontier or the field, it may be paid on the order of the commanding officer, not to exceed the regulated amount, by a medical disbursing officer, or a quartermaster.

1309. When medical attendance is required by officers or enlisted men on service, or for the authorized servants of such officers, and the attendance of a medical officer cannot be had, the officer, or, if there be no officer, then the enlisted man, may employ a private physician and a just account therefor will be paid by the medical bureau.

1310. The account will set out the name of the patient, the date of and charge for each visit and for medicines. The physician will make a certificate to the account in case of an officer, or affidavit in the case of an enlisted man, that the account is correct, and the charges are the customary charges of the place.

1311. The officer will make his certificate, or the enlisted man his affidavit, to the correctness of the account, that he was on service at the place, and stating the circumstances preventing him from receiving the services of a medical officer.

1312. When the charge is against an officer, he will pay the account if practicable, and transmit it to the medical bureau for reimbursement; in all other cases the account will be transmitted to the medical bureau for settlement.

1313. If the charge is against a deceased officer or enlisted man, the physician will make the affidavit, before required, to the account, and that he has been paid no part of it.

1314. No charges for consultation fees will be paid by the medical bureau, nor will any account for medical attendance or medicines be paid, if the officer or enlisted man be not on service.

1315. A board of not less than three medical officers will be appointed from time to time by the Secretary of War, to examine applicants for appointment of assistant-surgeons, and assistant-surgeons for promotion. And no one shall be so appointed or promoted until so examined and found qualified.

1316. The board will scrutinize rigidly the moral habits, professional acquirements, and physical qualifications of the candidates, and report favorably, either for appointment or promotion, in no case admitting of a reasonable doubt.

1317. The Secretary of War will designate the applicants to be examined for appointment of assistant-surgeon. They must be between 21 and 28 years of age. The board will report their respective merits in the several branches of the examination, and their relative merit from the whole; agreeably whereto, if vacancies happen within two years thereafter, they will receive appointments and take rank in the medical corps.

1318. When an assistant-surgeon has served five years, he is subject to be examined for promotion. If he decline the examination, or be found not qualified by moral habits or professional acquirements, he ceases to be a medical officer of the army.

1319. An applicant for appointment failing at one examination, may be allowed a second, after two years: but never a third.

1320. Medical Cadets will be selected, from among the applicants who have been examined and approved by a Medical Board, by the Surgeon-General, who will assign them to duty at such places and in such numbers as the service may require. These candidates will be enlisted for the full term, by the Surgeon-General, or by a medical officer of the army authorized by him, who will at once cause to be administered to the Cadet the following oath:

I, —— ——, appointed a —— in the army of the United States, do solemnly swear, or affirm, that I will bear true allegiance to the United States of America, and that I will serve them honestly and faithfully against all their enemies or opposers whatsoever; and observe and obey the orders of the President of the United States, and the orders of the officers appointed over me, according to the rules and articles for the government of the armies of the United States.

Sworn to and subscribed before me, at ——, this —— day of——, 186

—— ——, *Justice of the Peace.*

1321. Medical Cadets will have the rank and pay of the Cadets at the Military Academy, and be under the direction and control of medical officers alone. They will be entitled each to one room as quarters, and fuel therefor, as allowed a Sergeant-Major, and will take choice next after Brevet Second Lieutenants in the selection of quarters. Transportation will be allowed them as in cases of paymasters' clerks.

1322. On the fifteenth day of the last month of his term of service, each Medical Cadet will report the fact to the medical officer in charge, whose duty it is to report the same to the Surgeon-General, together with a report of the general character and competency of the Cadet.

1323. The Secretary of War will appoint from the enlisted men of the army, or cause to be enlisted, as many competent hospital stewards as the service may require, not to exceed one for each post.

1324. The senior medical officer of a hospital requiring a steward may recommend a competent non-commissioned officer or soldier to be appointed, which recommendation the commanding officer shall forward to the Adjutant-General of the army, with his remarks thereon, and with the remarks of the company commander. And, as the object of these more permanent appointments is to procure the services of a more competent body of hospital stewards, no soldier nor citizen must henceforth be recommended for appointment who is not *known* to be temperate, honest, and in every way reliable, as well as sufficiently intelligent, and skilled in pharmacy, for the proper discharge of the responsible duties likely to be devolved upon him.

1325. When no competent enlisted man can be procured, the medical officer will report the fact to the Surgeon-General.* Applications and testimonials of competency, from persons seeking to be enlisted for hospital stewards, may be addressed to the Surgeon-General.

1326. The commanding officer may re-enlist a hospital steward at the expiration of his term of service, on the recommendation of the medical officer.

1327. Hospital stewards, whenever stationed in places whence no post return is made to the Adjutant-General's office, or when on furlough, will, at the end of every month, report themselves by letter to the Adjutant-General and Surgeon-General, as well as to the medical director of the military department in which they may be serving; to each of whom they will also report each new assignment to duty, or change of station, ordered in their case, noting carefully the number, date, and source of the order directing the same. They will likewise report monthly, when on furlough, to the medical officer in charge of the hospital to which they are attached.

---

* The current wants of the service may, however, be supplied by a detail from the command, on the recommendation of the medical officer, of a soldier to act as temporary steward, thus affording the means of a careful probation of all soldiers so detailed, who are ambitious of one day deserving a permanent appointment. Stewards thus detailed at posts, or with a body of troops of more than four companies, will receive the pay and allowances of a sergeant of ordnance; and at all other posts, or with smaller bodies of troops, the pay and allowances of a first sergeant of infantry. (See Act July 5, 1838.)

1328. The accounts of pay, clothing, &c., of hospital stewards must be kept by the medical officers under whose immediate direction they are serving, who are also responsible for certified statements of such accounts, and correct descriptive lists of such stewards, to accompany them in case of transfer—as, also, that their final statements and certificates of discharge are accurately made out, when they are at length discharged from service.

AMBULANCES.

1329. The following amount and kind of transportation for the sick and wounded may be provided for troops on marches and in campaigns against Indians:

1. For commands of less than five companies, to each company, one two-wheeled ambulance.
2. For a battalion, of five companies, one four-wheeled and five two-wheeled ambulances.
3. For a regiment, two four-wheeled and ten two-wheeled ambulances.

1330. The following schedule of transports for the sick and wounded and for hospital supplies will be adopted for a state of war with a civilized enemy:

1. For commands of less than three companies, one two-wheeled transport cart for hospital supplies, and to each company one two-wheeled ambulance.
2. For commands of more than three and less than five companies, two two-wheeled transport carts, and to each company one two-wheeled ambulance.
3. For a battalion of five companies, one four-wheeled ambulance, five two-wheeled ambulances, and two two-wheeled transport carts. For each additional company less than ten, one two-wheeled transport cart.
4. For a regiment of ten companies, two four-wheeled ambulances, ten two-wheeled ambulances, and four two-wheeled transport carts; and for greater commands in proportion.

1331. Ambulances will not be used for any other than the specific purpose for which they are designed, viz. the transportation of the sick and wounded; and those hereafter provided for the army, will be made according to a pattern to be furnished the Quartermaster's Department by the Surgeon-General.

1332. The transport carts must be made after the models of the two-wheeled ambulances (their interior arrangement for the sick excepted), and to have solid board flooring to the body.

1333. Horse-litters may be prepared and furnished to posts whence they may be required for service on ground not admitting the employment of two-wheeled carriages; said litters to be composed of a canvas bed similar to the present stretcher, and of two poles each sixteen feet long, to be made in sections, with head and foot-pieces constructed to act as stretchers to keep the poles apart.

1334. The allowance of hospital attendants in the field will be, for one company, one steward, one nurse, and one cook; for each additional company, one nurse; and for commands of over five companies, one additional cook.

HOSPITAL TENTS.

1335. Hospital tents must in future be made according to the pattern of the present tent and of the same material, but smaller, and having on one end a lapel so as to admit of two or more tents being joined and thrown into one with a continuous covering or roof. The dimensions to be these: In length, 14 feet; in width, 15 feet; in height (centre), 11 feet, with a wall $4\frac{1}{2}$ feet, and a "fly" of appropriate size. The ridge-pole to be made in two sections after the present pattern; and to measure 14 feet when joined. Such a tent will accommodate from 8 to 10 patients comfortably.

1336. The following will be the allowance of tents for the sick, their attendants and hospital supplies:

COMMANDS.	HOSPITAL TENTS.	SIBLEY TENTS.	COMMON TENTS.
For one company	..	1	1
For three companies	1	1	1
For five companies	2	1	1
For seven companies	2	1	1
For ten companies	3	1	1

1337. Upon the march or in battle, medical officers will habitually be attended by an orderly, carrying a hospital knapsack. This knapsack to be made of light wood and of the ordinary size; to be divided into four compartments or drawers, and to be covered with canvas or other suitable material; the object being to carry in an accessible shape such instruments, dressings, and medicines as may be needed in an emergency on the march or in the field.

PART III.

GENERAL ORDERS RELATIVE TO THE MEDICAL DEPARTMENT.

GENERAL ORDERS NO. 6.

War Department, Adjutant-General's Office,
Washington, *March* 13, 1861.

The uniform, dress, and horse equipments of the army having been changed in many respects since the General Regulations of 1857, the following description of them is published for the information of all concerned:

COAT.

1. All officers shall wear a frock coat of dark blue cloth, the skirt to extend two-thirds to three-fourths of the distance from the top of the hip to the bend of the knee; single-breasted for captains and lieutenants, double-breasted for all other grades.

BUTTONS.

18. For officers of the general staff—gilt, convex, with spread eagle and stars, and plain borders; large size, seven-eighths of an inch in exterior diameter; small size, one half inch.

TROWSERS.

26. For officers of the general staff—dark-blue cloth with a gold cord, one-eighth of an inch in diameter, along the outer seam.

HAT AND TRIMMINGS.

32. For officers—of best black felt. The dimensions of medium size to be as follows: Width of brim, 3¼ inches; height of crown, 6¼ inches; oval of tip, ½ inch; taper of crown, ¾ inch; curve of head, ⅜ inch; the binding to be ½ inch deep of best black-ribbed silk; silk and gold cord with acorn ends; the rim of the hat fasten-

ed up on the right side with an eagle attached to the side; three black ostrich feathers on the left side; a gold embroidered wreath in front, on black velvet ground, encircling the letters U. S. in silver—old English characters.

SASH.

60. For officers of the medical department—medium or emerald green silk net, with silk bullion fringe ends.

SHOULDER STRAPS.

For officers of the general staff—dark-blue cloth, one and three-eighth inches wide by four inches long; bordered with an embroidery of gold, one-fourth of an inch wide. For majors—one gold embroidered wreath at each end. For a captain—two bars placed parallel to each other at each end. For a first lieutenant—one bar at each end.

GENERAL ORDERS NO. 8.

War Department, Adjutant-General's Office,
Washington, *April* 3, 1861.

PROMOTIONS—MEDICAL DEPARTMENT.

Asst.-Surgeon Lewis A. Edwards to be Surgeon, February 19, 1864, *vice* De Leon, resigned.

Asst.-Surgeon John F. Hammond to be Surgeon, February 25, 1861, *vice* Moore, resigned.

RESIGNED.

Surgeon Samuel P. Moore, February 25, 1861.
Surgeon David C. De Leon, February 19, 1861.
Asst.-Surgeon George K. Wood, January 1, 1861.
Asst.-Surgeon William A. Carswell, March 25, 1861.
Asst.-Surgeon James H. Berrien, March 17, 1861.

GENERAL ORDERS NO. 15.

War Department, Adjutant-General's Office,
Washington, *May* 4, 1861.

Plan of Organization of the Volunteer Forces in the Service of the United States by the President:

Infantry—Each regiment will be organized as follows: One Assistant-Surgeon, one Hospital Steward.

Regiment of Cavalry—One Assistant-Surgeon, one Hospital Steward.

Each Brigade will consist of: one Surgeon.

GENERAL ORDERS NO. 16.

War Department, Adjutant-General's Office,
Washington, *May* 4, 1861.

Plan of Organization for Increase of the Force of the Regular Army:

Infantry, each battalion—One Hospital Steward.
Cavalry, each battalion—One Hospital Steward.
Artillery, each regiment—One Hospital Steward.

GENERAL ORDERS NO. 20.

War Department, Adjutant-General's Office,
Washington, *May* 14, 1864.

2. There will be added to the medical department of the army, ten Surgeons and twenty Assistant-Surgeons.

The Surgeons will be promoted according to existing laws and regulations from the senior Assistant-Surgeons; and the Assistant-Surgeons will be appointed from civil life after having passed the usual examination by a Board from the Medical Department of the army.

Due public notice of the appointment and time and place of meeting of the Board will be given.

GENERAL ORDERS NO. 23.

War Department, Adjutant-General's Office,
Washington, *May* 20, 1861.

It is with pain that the Secretary of War announces to the service the loss of a distinguished veteran officer, the late Surgeon-General Thomas Lawson, of the Army, who died at Norfolk, Virginia, on the 15th instant.

Having in 1811 resigned from the Navy, where he had served two years, Dr. Lawson passed immediately into the Army, a service with which from that time he has been uninterruptedly connected. Full of a military fire which not even the frosts of age could quench, and of a zeal for the honor of his profession which made his administration of the Medical Department a model of inflexibility, efficiency, and economy, he never spared himself, and was always prompt to volunteer his services whenever they might be required. Thus, after having gone with credit through the war of 1812–15, he was one of the first to hasten with General Gaines to the relief of our forces in Florida, and having been placed at the head of a regiment of volunteers by the suffrages of the gallant Louisianians who composed it, he acquitted himself with much credit in this new sphere of duty, and proved himself an able and effective Colonel. In fact, so marked were the military traits in his character, and among those especially his personal intrepidity, that at the close of the Mexican war he was rewarded for his services in it by a brevet of Brigadier-General in the army.

As an appropriate tribute of respect to his memory, there will be fired at every military post on the day after the receipt of this order, eleven minute guns, commencing at meridian, and the national flag will be displayed at half-staff from the same hour until sunset of the same day, and for thirty days the prescribed badge of mourning will be worn by the officers of the army.

GENERAL ORDERS NO. 24.

War Department, Adjutant-General's Office,
Washington, *May* 22, 1861.

I. PROMOTIONS—MEDICAL DEPARTMENT.

Surgeon Clement A. Finley, to be Surgeon-General, May 15, 1861, *vice* Lawson, deceased.

Asst.-Surgeon Elisha J. Bailey, to be Surgeon, *vice* Finley promoted, May 15, 1861.

IV. CASUALTIES—RESIGNED.

Asst.-Surgeon Charles H. Smith, April 25, 1861.
Asst.-Surgeon John M. Haden, April 25, 1861.
Asst.-Surgeon Edward W. Johns, April 22, 1861.
Asst.-Surgeon William W. Anderson, April 20, 1861.
Asst.-Surgeon Elisha P. Langworthy, April 30, 1861.
Asst.-Surgeon Andrew J. Foard, April 1, 1861.
Asst.-Surgeon Richard Potts, May 7, 1861.
Asst.-Surgeon Robert L. Brodie, May 7, 1861.
Asst.-Surgeon Nathaniel S. Crowell, May 17, 1861.
Asst.-Surgeon William J. L. Engle, April 30, 1861.
Asst.-Surgeon Asa Wall, May 11, 1861.
Asst.-Surgeon Charles Brewer, May 7, 1861.
Asst.-Surgeon Archibald M. Fauntleroy, May 9, 1861.

DIED.

Brevet Brigadier-General Thomas Lawson, Surgeon-General, at Norfolk, Virginia, May 15, 1861.

GENERAL ORDERS NO. 25.

War Department, Adjutant-General's Office,
Washington, *May* 25, 1861.

The plan of organization for the Volunteer Forces designated in General Orders No. 15 of May 4, 1861, is so modified as to allow one surgeon and one assistant-surgeon to each regiment, to be appointed by the Governors of the respective States, after having passed an examination by a competent Medical Board appointed by the Governors of the States. The appointments to be subject to the approval of the Secretary of War.

GENERAL ORDERS NO. 31.

War Department, Adjutant-General's Office,
Washington, *June* 9, 1861.

Women nurses will not reside in the camps, nor accompany regiments on a march; but those who apply for service and are highly accredited, having certificates from two physicians and two clergymen of standing, and will forward the same to Miss D. L. Dix at Washington, will receive a certificate in return, accrediting them for service in any military hospital of the United States where such services are required.

GENERAL ORDERS NO. 35.

War Department, Adjutant-General's Office,
Washington, *June* 20, 1861.

2. The several Medical Directors of the army will, when they have reason to doubt the professional competency of any of the medical officers under their charge, organize a Board of not less than three medical officers, who shall examine said officers of questioned professional capacity, and decide whether they are competent to the performance of their duties.

GENERAL ORDERS NO. 39.

War Department, Adjutant-General's Office,
Washington, *July* 1, 1861.

1. No volunteer will be discharged upon surgeon's certificate of disability until the certificate shall have been submitted to the Medical Director, and shall have been approved and countersigned by him.

GENERAL ORDERS NO. 46.

War Department, Adjutant-General's Office,
Washington, *July* 19, 1861.

4. Brigade-Surgeons rank as Surgeons only.

GENERAL ORDERS NO. 48.

War Department, Adjutant-General's Office,
Washington, *July* 31, 1861.

1. The following Act of Congress is published for the information of all concerned:

An Act to Increase the present Military Establishment of the United States.

Be it enacted by the Senate and House of Representatives of the United States of America in Congress assembled: That there shall be added to the regular army as now authorized by law, nine regiments of infantry, one regiment of cavalry, and one regiment of artillery.

SEC. 2. *And be it further enacted*, That the field and staff commissioned and non-commissioned officers of the regiments hereinbefore authorized, shall be as follows:

To each regiment of Infantry—One Hospital Steward.
To each battalion of Cavalry—One Hospital Steward.
To the regiment of Artillery—One Hospital Steward.

GENERAL ORDERS NO. 49.

War Department, Adjutant-General's Office,
Washington, *August* 3, 1861.

1. The following Acts of Congress are published for the information of the army:

AN ACT to authorize the Employment of Volunteers to aid in Enforcing the Laws and protecting Public Property.

SEC. 3. Each brigade shall have one Surgeon.

Each regiment of Infantry shall have one Surgeon, one Assistant Surgeon, and one Hospital Steward.

GENERAL ORDERS NO. 51.

War Department, Adjutant General's Office,
Washington, *August* 3, 1861.

1. Hereafter, whenever volunteers are mustered into the service of the United States, they will at the same time be minutely examined by the surgeon and assistant-surgeon of the regiments, to ascertain whether they have the physical qualifications necessary for the military service. The certificate given by the surgeon (in case of rejected recruit—ED.) will in all cases state whether the disability existed prior to the date of muster, or was contracted after it.

GENERAL ORDERS NO. 54.

War Department, Adjutant-General's Office,
Washington, *August* 10, 1864.

1. The following Acts of Congress are published for the information of the army:

AN ACT providing for the better Organization of the Military Establishment.

SEC. 5. *And be it further enacted*, That there be added to the medical staff of the army, a corps of medical cadets, whose duty it shall be to act as dressers in the general hospitals and as ambulance attendants in the field, under the direction and control of the medical officers alone. They shall have the same rank and pay as the military cadets at West Point. Their number shall be regulated by the exigencies of the service, at no time to exceed fifty. It shall be composed of young men of liberal education, students of medicine, between the ages of eighteen and twenty-three, who have been reading medicine for two years, and have attended at least one course of lectures in a medical college. They shall enlist for one year, and be subject to the rules and articles of war. On the fifteenth day of the last month of their service the near approach of their discharge shall be reported to the Surgeon-General, in order, if desired, that they may be relieved by another detail of applicants.

Sec. 6. *And be it further enacted*, That in general or permanent hospitals, female nurses may be substituted for soldiers, when in the opinion of the Surgeon-General or medical officer in charge, it is expedient to do so, the number of female nurses to be indicated by the Surgeon-General or surgeon in charge of the hospital. The nurses so employed shall receive forty cents a day and one ration in kind or by commutation, in lieu of all emoluments except transportation in kind.

Sec. 13. *And be it further enacted*, That the army ration shall be increased as follows, viz.: Twenty ounces of bread or flour, or one pound of hard bread instead of the present issue; fresh beef shall be issued as often as the commanding officer of any detachment or regiment shall require it, when practicable, in place of salt meat; beans and rice and hominy shall be issued in the same ration, in the portions now provided by the regulations, and one pound of potatoes per man shall be issued at least three times a week if practicable; and when these articles cannot be issued in these proportions, an equivalent in value shall be issued in some other proper food, and a ration of tea may be substituted for a ration of coffee, upon the requisition of the proper officer: *Provided*, That after the present insurrection shall cease, the ration shall be as provided by law and regulations on the first day of July, 1861.

Sec. 14. *And be it further enacted*, That there may be allowed in hospitals, to be provided under such rules as the Surgeon-General of the army, with the approval of the Secretary of War, may prescribe, such quantities of fresh or preserved fruits, milk or butter, and of eggs, as may be necessary for the proper diet of the sick.

GENERAL ORDERS NO. 59.

War Department, Adjutant-General's Office,
Washington, *August* 17, 1864.

1. So much of paragraph 3, of Special Orders No. 185, from this office, dated July 12, 1861, as relates to the allowances of female nurses employed in Permanent and General Hospitals, is hereby rescinded; and such persons will receive, from and after the 3d inst., 40 cents per day and one ration in kind or by commutation, at cost price, in lieu of all emoluments except transportation in kind.

3. Every officer of the army will immediately report his address to this office, and thereafter every change of address, no matter whether permanent or temporary.

GENERAL ORDERS NO. 62.

War Department, Adjutant-General's Office,
Washington, *August* 20, 1861.

Appointments made by the President in the Volunteer Force raised in Conformity with Proclamation of May 3, 1863.

MEDICAL DEPARTMENT, BRIGADE SURGEONS, AUGUST 3, 1861.

George H. Lyman, of Mass.
F. H. Hamilton, of New York.
Henry S. Hewitt, of New York.
J. H. Brinton, of Penn.
John A. Lydell, of New York.
John C. Dalton, of New York.
George Suckley, of New York.
Henry Bryant, of Mass.
P. W. Ellsworth, of Conn.
Luther V. Bell, of Mass.
S. W. Gross, of Penn.
David Prince, of Illinois.
A. H. Hoff, of New York.
W. H. Church, of New York.
Joseph W. Freer, of Illinois.
Rufus H. Gilbert, of New York.
J. E. Quidor, of New Jersey.
Charles McMillan, of New York.
Charles O'Leary, of Ohio.
J. G. F. Holston, of the District of Columbia.
A. B. Campbell, of Penn.
J. V. Z. Blaney, of Illinois.
Thomas Sim, of Illinois.
J. S. Bobbs, of Indiana.
Peter Pineo, of Mass.
W. E. Waters, of District of Columbia.
O. Martin, of Mass.
J. H. Rauch, of Illinois.
William D. Stewart, of Indiana.
N. R. Derby, of Penn.
Daniel McRuer, of Maine.
S. R. Haven, of Illinois.
A. E. Stocker, of Penn.
J. Owen, of Penn.
W. C. Thompson, of Indiana.

AUGUST 5, 1861.

James King, of Penn.
T. Rush Spencer, of New York,
J. D. Robinson, of Ohio.
William Clendenin, of Ohio.
George G. Shumard, of Ohio.

GENERAL ORDERS NO. 63.

War Department, Adjutant-General's Office,
Washington, *August* 22, 1861.

1. * * Asst. Surgeon David P. Ramseur, U.S.A., having deserted to the enemy, is likewise dismissed the service, to date from the 17th inst.

GENERAL ORDERS NO. 64.

War Department, Adjutant-General's Office,
Washington, *August* 22, 1861.

PROMOTIONS.—MEDICAL DEPARTMENT.

Asst.-Surgeon George E. Cooper, to be Surgeon, May 21st, 1861, to fill an original vacancy.

Asst.-Surgeon Ebenezer Swift, to be Surgeon, May 21st, 1861, to fill an original vacancy.

Asst.-Surgeon Glover Perrin, to be Surgeon, May 21st, 1861, to fill an original vacancy.

Asst.-Surgeon Peter G. S. Ten Broeck, to be Surgeon, May 21st, 1861, to fill an original vacancy.

Asst.-Surgeon John Campbell, to be Surgeon, May 21st, 1861, to fill an original vacancy.

Asst.-Surgeon John E. Summers, to be Surgeon, May 21st, 1861, to fill an original vacancy.

Asst.-Surgeon Charles H. Crane, to be Surgeon, May 21st, 1861, to fill an original vacancy.

Asst.-Surgeon Lyman H. Stone, to be Surgeon, May 21st, 1861, to fill an original vacancy.

Asst.-Surgeon Thomas A. McParlin, to be Surgeon, May 21st, 1861, to fill an original vacancy.

Asst.-Surgeon William F. Edgar, to be Surgeon, May 21st, 1861, to fill an original vacancy.

Asst.-Surgeon Joseph B. Brown, to be Surgeon, July 4th, 1861, vice Simpson, deceased.

APPOINTMENTS.

William A. Hammond, of Maryland, to be Asst.-Surgeon, *vice* Wood, resigned, to date from May 28, 1861.

Joseph P. Wright, of Pennsylvania, to be Asst.-Surgeon, *vice* Edwards, promoted, to date from May 28, 1861.

Havilah M. Sprague, of Connecticut, to be Asst.-Surgeon, *vice* Hammond, promoted, to date from May 28, 1861.

Charles C. Gray, of New York, to be Asst.-Surgeon, *vice* Berrien, resigned, to date May 28, 1861.

William C. Spencer, to be Asst.-Surgeon, *vice* Carswell, resigned, to date May 28, 1861.

Francis L. Town, of Pennsylvania, to be Assist.-Surgeon, *vice* Foard, resigned, to date May 28, 1861.

Alexander Ingraham, of Ohio, to be Asst.-Surgeon, *vice* Anderson, resigned, to date May 28, 1861.

Peter V. Schenck, of New Jersey, to be Asst.-Surgeon, *vice* Johns, resigned, to date from May 28, 1861.

John W. S. Gouley, of New York, to be Asst.-Surgeon, *vice* Smith, resigned, to date from May 28, 1861.

Dallas Bache, of Pennsylvania, to be Asst.-Surgeon, *vice* Haden, resigned, to date from May 28, 1861.

Blencowe E. Fryer, of Pennsylvania, to be Asst.-Surgeon, *vice* Langworthy, resigned, to date from May 28, 1861.

John H. Frantz, of Maryland, to be Asst.-Surgeon, *vice* L'Engle, resigned, to date from May 28, 1861.

Webster Lindsley, of the District of Columbia, to be Asst.-Surgeon, *vice* Potts, resigned, to date from May 28, 1861.

Charles E. Goddard, of New York, to be Asst.-Surgeon, *vice* Brodie, resigned, to date from May 28, 1861.

Henry R. Silliman, of Pennsylvania, to be Asst.-Surgeon, *vice* Brewer, resigned, to date from May 28, 1861.

Philip C. Davis, of the District of Columbia, to be Asst.-Surgeon, *vice* Fauntleroy, resigned, to date from May, 28, 1861.

Joseph S. Smith, of the District of Columbia, to be Asst.-Surgeon, *vice* Wall, resigned, to date from May 28, 1861.

Charles J. Wilson, of the District of Columbia, to be Asst.-Surgeon, *vice* Crowell, resigned, to date from May 28, 1861.

James F. Weeds, of Ohio, to be Asst.-Surgeon, *vice* Bailey, promoted, to date from May 28, 1861.

Charles B. White, of New York, to be Asst.-Surgeon, *vice* Swift, promoted, to date from May 28, 1862.

George M. Sternberg, of New York, to be Asst.-Surgeon, *vice* Cooper, promoted, to date from May 28, 1861.

Lawrence H. Sheldon, of Connecticut, to be Asst.-Surgeon, *vice* Perin, promoted, to date from July 26, 1861.

Joseph J. Woodward, of Pennsylvania, to be Asst. Surgeon, *vice* Ten Broeck, promoted, to date from August 5, 1861.

Edward S. Dunster, of New York, to be Asst.-Surgeon, *vice* Campbell, promoted, to date from August 5, 1861.

Elias J. Marsh, of New Jersey, to be Asst.-Surgeon, *vice* Summers, promoted, to date from August 5, 1861.

Robert F. Weir, of New York, to be Asst.-Surgeon, *vice* Crane, promoted, to date from August 5, 1861.

Thomas C. Brainerd, of Pennsylvania, to be Asst.-Surgeon, *vice* McParlin, promoted, to date from August 5, 1861.

Morris J. Asch, of Pennsylvania, to be Asst.-Surgeon, *vice* McParlin, promoted, to date from August 5, 1861.

Henry S. Schell, of Pennsylvania, to be Asst.-Surgeon, *vice* Guild, dismissed, to date from August 5, 1861.

Charles K. Winne, of New York, to be Asst.-Surgeon, *vice* Edgar, promoted, to date from August 5, 1861.

Joseph E. Semple, of New York, to be Asst.-Surgeon, *vice* Williams, resigned, to date from August 5, 1861.

William H. Forwood, of Pennsylvania, to be Asst.-Surgeon, *vice* Brown, promoted, to date from August 5, 1861.

James H. Pooley, of New York, to be Asst.-Surgeon, August 5, 1861, to fill an original vacancy.

Ely McClellan, of Pennsylvania, to be Asst.-Surgeon, August 5, 1861, to fill an original vacancy.

Charles A. McCall, of Pennsylvania, to be Asst.-Surgeon, August 5, 1861, to fill an original vacancy.

Samuel A. Storrow, of the District of Columbia, to be Asst.-Surgeon, August 5, 1861, to fill an original vacancy.

John C. C. Downing, of the District of Columbia, to be Asst.-Surgeon, August 5, 1861, to fill an original vacancy.

William D. Wolverton, of New Jersey, to be Asst.-Surgeon, August 5, 1861, to fill an original vacancy.

Josiah F. Kennedy, of Iowa, to be Asst.-Surgeon, August 5, 1861, to fill an original vacancy.

John J. Butler, of the District of Columbia, to be Asst.-Surgeon, August 5, 1861, to fill an original vacancy.

William R. Ramsey, of Pennsylvania, to be Asst.-Surgeon, August 5, 1861, to fill an original vacancy.

Thomas H. Helsby, of Maryland, to be Asst.-Surgeon, August 5, 1861, to fill an original vacancy.

Albert Hartsuff, of Michigan, to be Asst.-Surgeon, August 5, 1861, to fill an original vacancy.

Charles R. Greenleaf, of Ohio, to be Asst.-Surgeon, August 5, 1861, to fill an original vacancy.

Philip Adolphus, of Maryland, to be Asst.-Surgeon, August 5, 1861, to fill an original vacancy.

Andrew J. Baxter, of Ohio, to be Asst.-Surgeon, August 5, 1861, to fill an original vacancy.

Bolivar Knickerbocker, of Pennsylvania, to be Asst.-Surgeon, August 5, 1861, to fill an original vacancy.

Lewis M. Eastman, of Maryland, to be Asst.-Surgeon, August 5, 1861, to fill an original vacancy.

Johnson V. Middleton, of the District of Columbia, to be Asst.-Surgeon, August 5, 1861, to fill an original vacancy.

William Thomson, of Pennsylvania, to be Asst.-Surgeon, August 5, 1861, to fill an original vacancy.

RESIGNED.

Asst.-Surgeon Thomas H. Williams, June 1, 1861.
Asst.-Surgeon Rodney Glisan, June 7, 1861.
Asst.-Surgeon Aquila T. Ridgeley, June 23, 1861.
Asst.-Surgeon Edward N. Covey, June 1, 1861
Asst.-Surgeon John J. Gaenslen, August 17, 1861.

DIED.

Surgeon Richard F. Simpson, at Key West Barracks, Florida, July 4, 1861.
Asst.-Surgeon Calvin G. Hollenbush, at McKey's Half Falls, Pa., August 6, 1861.

DISMISSED.

Asst.-Surgeon Lafayette Guild, July 1, 1861.
Asst.-Surgeon David P. Ramseur, August 17, 1861.

GENERAL ORDERS No. 68.

War Department, Adjutant-General's Office,
Washington, *August* 27, 1861.

APPOINTMENTS.—MEDICAL DEPARTMENT.

To be Asst.-Surgeons to date from August 26, 1861:

John Bell, of New Hampshire, to fill an original vacancy.

John H. Janeway, of Pennsylvania, to fill an original vacancy.
Henry A. Dubois, of New York, *vice* Williams, resigned.
Benjamin Howard, of New York, *vice* Glisan, resigned.
Henry C. Parry, of Pennsylvania, *vice* Ridgely, resigned.
Henry R. Tilton, of New Jersey, *vice* Gaenslen, resigned.
Samuel M. Horton, of Pennsylvania, *vice* Covey, resigned.
John C. G. Happerseth, of Pennsylvania, *vice* Hollenbush, resigned.

GENERAL ORDERS No. 75.

War Department, Adjutant-General's Office,
Washington, *September* 11, 1861.

The following order has been received from the War Department, and is published for the information of all concerned:

War Department, September 9, 1861.

For the purpose of preserving accurate and permanent records of deceased soldiers, and their place of burial, it is hereby ordered that the Quartermaster-General of the U. S. Army, shall cause to be printed and placed in every General and Post Hospital of the army, blank books and forms for preserving said records. The Quartermaster will also provide proper means for a registered head-board, to be secured at the head of each soldier's grave as directed in the following special order to Commanding Officers in reference to the interment of deceased soldiers.

It is hereby ordered that, whenever any soldier or officer of the U. S. Army dies, it shall be the duty of the Commanding Officer of the military corps or department in which such person dies, to cause the regulations and forms provided in the foregoing directions to the Quartermaster-General to be properly executed.

It is also ordered that any Adjutant, Acting-Adjutant (or Commander), of a military post or company, immediately upon reception of any mortuary record from a military company, shall transmit the same to the Adjutant-General at Washington.

GENERAL ORDERS No. 98.

War Department, Adjutant-General's Office,
Washington, *November* 13, 1861.

2. The insane of the military service are entitled to treatment in the Government Hospital established in this city. To protect, however, their own interests, as well as those of the Government, it is prescribed by the Secretary of War, that to procure admission into the hospital, application must be made to the Adjutant-General, setting forth the name, rank, company, and regiment of the patient, with a certificate from the surgeon of the regiment as to the duration of the insanity, and whether insane before enlistment. It will likewise be accompanied by the descriptive list of the soldier, and copies of his pay and clothing account. The application should precede the arrival of the soldier in this city by at least one day, that the signature of the Secretary of War may be obtained to the paper, authorizing admission into the hospital, and that the patient may not have to wait in the streets during that time.

On the departure of the patient from his station, the Commanding Officer will give such orders to the person in charge as will provide for the transportation of the necessary attendants to the institution and back again to their post, and for their subsistence, either in kind or by commutation, during their absence.

To procure the release of a patient, when cured, or for delivery to his friends, application must again be made to the Adjutant-General, who will procure the necessary authorization, and also cause a statement of his accounts to be made and delivered to him.

GENERAL ORDERS No. 102.

Head-Quarters of the Army, Adjutant-General's Office,
Washington, *November* 25, 1861.

4. The uniform for Chaplains of the army, will be plain black frock coat with standing collar, and one row of nine black buttons, plain black pantaloons, black felt hat, or army forage cap, without ornament. On occasions of ceremony a plain chapeau de bras may be worn.

GENERAL ORDERS No. 103.

Head-Quarters of the Army, Adjutant-General's Office,
Washington, *December* 4, 1861.

1. Asst.-Surgeon James C. Herndon, Medical Dept., U. S. Army, having left his post without leave, the President directs that he be dropped from the rolls of the army from November 27, 1861.

GENERAL ORDERS No. 106.

Head-Quarters of the Army, Adjutant-General's Office,
Washington, *December* 5, 1861.

PROMOTIONS.—MEDICAL DEPARTMENT.

Asst.-Surgeon Alexander B. Hasson, to be Surgeon, August 17, 1861, vice Madison, resigned.

APPOINTMENTS.

Alfred A. Woodhull, of Kansas, to be Asst.-Surgeon, September 19, 1861, vice Hasson, promoted.

William A. Bradley, of the District of Columbia, to be Asst.-Surgeon, to date from October 22, 1861, *vice* Crawford, appointed Major in the Thirteenth Infantry.

George P. Jaquett, of New Jersey, to be Asst.-Surgeon, to date from October 23, 1861, *vice* Ryland, deceased.

To be Brigade-Surgeons, to date September 4, 1861.

William Brodie, of Michigan; John T. Carpenter, of Pennsylvania; Alpheus B. Crosby, of New Hampshire; William Varian, of Illinois; O. M. Bryan, of Illinois; Tarrant A. Perkins, of Illinois; Thomas H. Bache, of Pennsylvania; James D. Strawbridge, of Pennsylvania; Josiah Curtis, of Massachusetts; F. N. Burke, of Ohio; D. W. Hartshorn, of Ohio; R. B. McCay, of Pennsylvania; W. W. Strew, of New York; John J. Craven, of New

Jersey; Robert L. Stanford, of Tennessee; A. P. Meylert, of Pennsylvania; Edwin Bentley, of Connecticut; S. L. Herrick, of Michigan; G. C. Blackman, of Ohio; R. B. Bontecou, of New York; Samuel Everett, of Illinois; J. H. Warren, of Massachusetts; D. W. Bliss, of Michigan; H. P. Stearns, of Connecticut; G. W. Stipp, of Illinois; G. H. Oliver, of New York; Alexander N. Dougherty, of New Jersey; E. C. Franklin, of Missouri; Geo. S. Kemble, of Pennsylvania; Geo. H. Hubbard, of New Hampshire; D. W. Hand, of Minnesota; Rufus K. Brown, of New York; W. G. Lowman, of Pennsylvania; John T. Crawford, of Pennsylvania; Thomas Antisell, of the District of Columbia; John McNulty, of New York; Daniel Meeker, of Pennsylvania; Gilman Kimball, of Massachusetts; Gideon S. Palmer, of Maine; J. H. Taylor, of Pennsylvania; W. M. Chambers, of Illinois; J. H. Grove, of Pennsylvania; A. H. Thurston, of New York; O. A. Judson, of Pennsylvania; I. F. Azpell, of New York; C. C. Cox, of Maryland; Timothy Haynes, of New Hampshire; Gabriel Grant, of New Jersey; C. B. Chapman, of Wisconsin; J. G. Keenon, of Kentucky; W. H. Mussey, of Ohio; C. W. Jones, Delaware; George Burr, of New York; Robert Roskoton, of Illinois; George L. Pancoast, of Pennsylvania; N. R. Mosely, of New York; F. H. Gross, of Pennsylvania; D. G. McKibbin, of Pennsylvania; T. F. Perley, of Maine; Robert Nicolls, of Illinois; M. Goldsmith, of Kentucky; James H. Faris, of Illinois; J. B. Peale, of Pennsylvania; W. J. Duffee, of Pennsylvania; James Bryan, of Pennsylvania; J. H. Thompson, of New York; R. A. Christian, of Pennsylvania; A. R. Egbert, of New Jersey; C. F. H. Campbell, of Pennsylvania; William Hayes, of Pennsylvania.

GENERAL ORDERS NO. 1.

War Department, Adjutant-General's Office,
Washington, *January* 6, 1862.

1. Transportation by express agency, being liable to abuse and very expensive, is prohibited by the Secretary of War, on public account, except in case of great emergency.

GENERAL ORDERS NO. 22.

War Department, Adjutant-General's Office,
Washington, *March* 1, 1862.

An Act making Additional Appropriations for the Support of the Army, for the Year ending June 30, 1862.

For the Medical and Hospital Department, one million of dollars.

GENERAL ORDERS NO. 36.

War Department, Adjutant-General's Office,
Washington, *April* 7, 1862.

1. The General Hospitals are under the direction of the Surgeon-General. Orders not involving expense of transportation may be given by him to transfer Medical Officers or Hospital

Stewards from one General Hospital to another, as he may deem best for the service.

2. The Chief Medical Officer to whom the charge of all the General Hospitals in a city may be entrusted, will cause certificates of disability to be made out for such men as, in his judgment, should be discharged. He will be responsible that the certificates are given for good cause, and that they are made in proper form, giving such medical description of the cases, with the degree of disability, as may enable the Pension Office to decide on any claim to pension which may be based upon them. The certificates of disability will be signed by the Chief Medical Officer and forwarded by him to the Military Commander in the city, who shall have authority to order the discharge and dispose of the case according to existing regulations.

3. The final statements, and all the discharge papers, will be made out under the supervision of the Military Commander, and signed by him. Where the men are provided with their descriptive rolls there will be no delay in discharging them after their certificates of disability are acted on. But if they have no descriptive rolls, application will be made to the Company Commander for the proper discharge papers, and the men may be maintained at the hospital a reasonable time while awaiting them, to avoid their being turned off without means of support. The discharge will, in all cases, bear the date when the papers are actually furnished the soldier.

4. When a man is received in any hospital without his descriptive roll, the fact will be immediately reported by the Medical Officer in charge to the Military Commander, who will at once call on the Company Commander, in the name of the Secretary of War, promptly to furnish the military history of the man, and his clothing, money, and other accounts with the Government.

5. When too long a delay would arise in discharging the man because of the remote station of his company, application will be made by the Medical Officer to the Adjutant-General for such account of the man as his records will furnish. To this partial descriptive roll the Medical Officer will add the period for which pay is due the man since his entry into the hospital. The man will then be discharged and receive the pay and travelling allowances thus shown to be due him, leaving the balance due him on account of clothing, retained pay, &c., for settlement in such manner as may hereafter be determined.

6. The Military Commander's duties, in reference to all troops and enlisted men who happen to come within the limits of his command, will be precisely those of a commanding officer of a military post.

7. It is made the duty of each Military Commander to correct, as far as may be in his power, the evils and irregularities arising from the peculiar state of the service at this time, by collecting stragglers and sending them forward to their proper stations, or

discharging them on certificates of disability, if, on examination by the Chief Medical Officer, they be found unfit for the service.

8. The Military Commander in each city will have control of such guards as may be furnished to preserve discipline and good order at the several military hospitals. He will advise the Adjutant-General of the army what number of companies will be required for such guards. He will cause them to be properly posted, relieved, and instructed.

9. Whenever the Chief Medical Officer shall report a number of patients as fit to join their regiments, the Military Commander will give the necessary orders to have them forwarded in good order and under suitable conduct.

10. The Chief Medical Officer in each city is authorized to employ as cooks, nurses, and attendants, any convalescent, wounded, or feeble men, who can perform such duties, instead of giving them discharges.

11. All officers and enlisted men of Volunteers who are on parole not to serve against the Rebels, will be considered on leave of absence, until notified of their exchange or discharge. They will immediately report their address to the Governors of their States, who will be duly informed from this office as to their exchange or discharge.

12. The duties of Military Commander, as above defined, will devolve, *in the District of Columbia*, on the Military Governor; *in the city of Baltimore*, on the Commander of the Middle Department; *in the city of Philadelphia*, on Lieutenant-Colonel H. Brooks, 2d Artillery, hereby assigned to that station; *in the city of New York*, and the military posts in that vicinity, on Brevet Brigadier General H. Brown, Colonel 5th United States Artillery.

By order of the Secretary of War:

L. THOMAS, *Adjutant-General.*

Adjutant-General's Office, *August* 26, 1862.

NOTE TO PAR. 5:

"In cases where too long a delay would arise in discharging a man because of the remote station of his Company," and when no descriptive lists, or partial descriptive list, can be obtained from this office, the men referred to will be discharged under this order, and an order given them on the Quartermaster's Department for transportation to their homes. This order will be signed by the same officer who signs the discharge. The Quartermaster's Department will furnish transportation to such men, upon the presentation of this order, requiring them also to show their discharge.

By order of Major-General Halleck:

E. D. TOWNSEND, *Assistant Adjutant-General.*

NOTE 2d TO PAR. 5:

The sentence "To this partial descriptive roll the Medical Officer will add the period for which pay is due the man since his entry into the hospital," will be understood to give him pay *on this final statement* from the muster *next preceding* his entry into the hospital until the date of his discharge.

GENERAL ORDERS NO 41.

War Department, Adjutant-General's Office,
Washington, *April* 16, 1862.

2. Transportation to soldiers on sick leave may be furnished and the cost stopped from their pay in the same manner as other stoppages are made.

GENERAL ORDERS NO 42.

War Department, Adjutant-General's Office,
Washington, *April* 16, 1862.

1. By direction of the President, Brigade-Surgeon J. H. Thompson, U. S. Vols., is hereby dismissed the service as an alarmist, on the recommendation of Major-General Burnside.

GENERAL ORDERS NO. 43.

War Department. Adjutant-General's Office,
Washington, *April* 19, 1862.

The following Act of Congress is published for the information of all concerned:

AN ACT to reorganize and increase the Efficiency of the Medical Department of the Army.

Be it enacted by the Senate and House of Representatives of the United States of America in Congress assembled, That there shall be added to the present Medical Corps of the Army, ten Surgeons and twenty Assistant-Surgeons, to be promoted and appointed under existing laws; twenty Medical Cadets, and as many Hospital Stewards as the Surgeon-General may consider necessary for the public service, and that their pay and that of all Hospital Stewards in the Volunteers as well as in the Regular Service, shall be thirty dollars per month, to be computed from the passage of this Act. And all Medical Cadets in the service shall, in addition to their pay, receive one ration per day, either in kind or commutation.

SEC. 2. *And be it further enacted,* That the Surgeon-General to be appointed under this Act shall have the rank, pay, and emoluments of a Brigadier-General. There shall be one Assistant Surgeon-General and one Medical Inspector-General of Hospitals, each with the rank, pay, and emoluments of a Colonel of Cavalry; and the Medical Inspector-General shall have, under the direction of the Surgeon-General, the supervision of all that relates to the sanitary condition of the Army, whether in transports, quarters, or camps, and of the hygiene, police, discipline, and efficiency of field and general hospitals, under such regulations as may be hereafter established.

SEC. 3. *And be it further enacted*, That there shall be eight Medical Inspectors with the rank, pay, and emoluments each of a Lieutenant-Colonel of Cavalry, and who shall be charged with the duty of inspecting the sanitary condition of transports, quarters, and camps of field and general hospitals, and who shall report to the Medical Inspector-General, under such regulations as may be hereafter established, all circumstances relating to the sanitary condition and wants of troops and of hospitals, and to the skill, efficiency, and good conduct of the officers and attendants connected with the Medical Department.

SEC. 4. *And be it further enacted*, That the Surgeon-General, the Assistant Surgeon-General, Medical Inspector-General and Medical Inspectors, shall, immediately after the passage of this Act, be appointed by the President, by and with the advice and consent of the Senate, by selection from the Medical Corps of the army, or from the Surgeons in the Volunteer service, without regard to their rank when so selected, but with sole regard to qualifications.

SEC. 5. *And be it further enacted*, That Medical Purveyors shall be charged, under the direction of the Surgeon-General, with the selection and purchase of all medical supplies, including new standard preparations, and of all books, instruments, hospital stores, furniture, and other articles required for the sick and wounded of the army. In all cases of emergency they may provide such additional accommodations for the sick and wounded of the army, and may transport such medical supplies as circumstances may render necessary, under such regulations as may hereafter be established, and shall make prompt and immediate issues upon all special requisitions made upon them under such circumstances by Medical Officers; and the special requisitions shall consist simply of a list of the articles required, the qualities required, dated and signed by the medical officers requiring them.

SEC. 6. *And be it further enacted*, That whenever the Inspector-General, or any one of the Medical Inspectors, shall report an officer of the Medical Corps disqualified, by age or otherwise, for promotion to a higher grade, or unfitted for the performance of his professional duties, he shall be reported by the Surgeon-General, for examination, to an Army Medical Board, as provided by the 17th section of the Act approved August 3, 1861.

SEC. 7. *And be it further enacted*, That the provisions of this act shall continue and be in force during the existence of the present rebellion, and no longer: *Provided, however*, That, when this act shall expire, all officers who shall have been promoted from the Medical Staff of the army under this act, shall retain their respective rank in the army, with such promotion as they would have been entitled to.

Approved April 16, 1862.

GENERAL ORDERS NO. 46.

War Department, Adjutant-General's Office,
Washington, *April* 23, 1862.

1. Surgeon-General Clement A. Finley, U. S. Army, having applied to be retired from active duty, after more than forty years' service, the President of the United States directs that his name be placed upon the list of retired officers, to date from April 14, 1862.

2. Surgeons from civil life who tender their services for the sick and wounded in the field, under the invitation of the Secretary of War, will each be allowed, while so employed, the use of a public horse, a tent, the necessary servants, and the privilege of purchasing subsistence stores from the Commissary Department.

GENERAL ORDERS NO. 47.

War Department, Adjutant-General's Office,
Washington, *April* 25, 1862.

When the care of sick and wounded soldiers is assumed by the States from which they came, the Subsistence Department will commute their ration at twenty-five cents.

GENERAL ORDERS NO. 48.

War Department, Adjutant-General's Office,
Washington, *April* 28, 1862.

1. Assistant-Surgeon William A. Hammond, U. S. Army, having been appointed by the President, Surgeon-General, with the rank of Brigadier-General, under the Act approved April 16, 1862, will enter without delay upon the duties of his office.

2. Applications for transportation for the removal of sick men, for nurses, and for supplies for the sick, will be made hereafter to the Surgeon-General. The Surgeon-General is also authorized to give passes at his discretion for private physicians, nurses, and friends of sick and wounded soldiers to attend and visit them.

GENERAL ORDERS NO. 51.

War Department, Adjutant-General's Office,
Washington, *May* 10, 1862.

I. Commanders of Departments will designate some officer in each city or town where there is a General Hospital, to perform the functions assigned to military commanders in "General Orders," No. 36.

II. When rations are commuted at twenty-five cents, under the provisions of "General Orders," No. 47, the physicians in charge of the State Hospitals will enter on their descriptive lists the dates between which the men have been subsisted.

III. When transportation is furnished to soldiers on sick leave, under paragraph II. of "General Orders," No. 41, the officers or surgeons of General Hospitals, who grant the furloughs, will note the cost of such transportation on the descriptive lists of the men.

Quartermasters will not hereafter pay bills for such transportation to the States.

GENERAL ORDERS NO. 53.

War Department, Adjutant-General's Office,
Washington, *May* 16, 1862.

The following acts of Congress are published for the information of all concerned:

II. An Act to facilitate the Discharge of Enlisted Men for Physical Disability.

Be it enacted by the Senate and House of Representatives of the United States of America in Congress assembled, That the Medical Inspector-General, or any Medical Inspector, is hereby authorized and empowered to discharge from the service of the United States any soldier or enlisted man, with the consent of such soldier or enlisted man, in the Permanent Hospitals, laboring under any physical disability which makes it disadvantageous to the service that he be retained therein, and the certificate, in writing, of such Inspector-General or Medical Inspector, setting forth the existence and nature of such physical disability, shall be sufficient evidence of such discharge: *Provided, however,* That every such certificate shall appear on its face to have been founded on personal inspection of the soldier so discharged, and shall specifically describe the nature and origin of such disability, and that such discharge shall be without prejudice to the right of such soldier or enlisted man to the pay due him at the date thereof, and report the same to the Adjutant-General and the Surgeon-General.

Approved May 14, 1862.

GENERAL ORDERS NO. 54.

War Department, Adjutant-General's Office,
Washington, *May* 17, 1862.

III. By direction of the President of the United States, Assistant-Surgeon J. J. Butler, U. S. Army, is hereby stricken from the rolls of the army.

GENERAL ORDERS NO. 55.

War Department, Adjutant-General's Office,
Washington, *May* 24, 1862.

I. The following Act of Congress is published for the information of all concerned:

An Act to authorize the Appointment of Medical Storekeepers and Chaplains of Hospitals.

Be it enacted by the Senate and House of Representatives of the United States of America in Congress assembled, That the Secretary of War be authorized to add to the Medical Department of the army, Medical Storekeepers, not exceeding six in number, who shall have the pay and emoluments of military storekeepers in the quartermaster's department, who shall be skilled apothecaries or druggists, who shall give the bond and security required by existing laws for military storekeepers in the quartermaster's department, and who shall be stationed at such points as the necessities of the army may require: *Provided*, That the provisions of this act shall remain in force only during the continuance of the present rebellion.

SEC. 2. *And be it further enacted*, That the President of the United States is hereby authorized to appoint, if he shall deem it necessary, a Chaplain for each Permanent Hospital, whose pay, with that of chaplains of hospitals heretofore appointed by him, shall be the same as that of regimental chaplains in the volunteer force; and who shall be subject to such rules in relation to leave of absence from duty as are prescribed for commissioned officers of the army.

Approved May 20, 1862.

II. The following are the Regulations which will govern the appointment of Medical Storekeepers under the first section of the foregoing act of Congress:

1. A Board of not less than three medical officers will be assembled by the Secretary of War to examine such applicants as may, by him, be authorized to appear before it.

2. Candidates, to be eligible to examination, shall be not less than 25 years, or more than 40 years of age; shall possess sufficient physical ability to perform their duties satisfactorily; and shall present with their applications satisfactory evidence of good moral character.

3. Candidates will be required to pass a satisfactory examination in the ordinary branches of a good English education, in pharmacy and materia medica; and to give proof that they possess the requisite business qualifications for the position.

4. The Board will report to the Secretary of War the relative merit of the candidates examined, and they will receive appointments accordingly.

5. When appointed, such Medical Storekeeper will be required to give a bond in the amount of $40,000 before he shall be allowed to enter upon the performance of his duties.

GENERAL ORDERS NO. 60.

War Department, Adjutant-General's Office,
Washington, *June* 6, 1862.

4. The principle being recognised that medical officers should not be held as prisoners of war, it is hereby directed that all medical officers so held by the United States shall be immediately and unconditionally discharged.

GENERAL ORDERS No. 61.

War Department, Adjutant-General's Office,
Washington, *June* 7, 1862.

The great number of officers absent from their regiments without sufficient cause is a serious evil which calls for immediate correction. By paragraph 177, General Regulations, the power of commanding officers to grant leaves of absence is limited to a "time of peace." In time of war leaves of absence will only be granted by the Secretary of War, except when the certificate of a medical officer shall show, beyond doubt, that a change of location "is necessary to save life, or prevent *permanent* disability." (*Paragraph* 186, *General Regulations.*) In such case, the Commander of an Army, a Department, or District, may grant not exceeding twenty days. At the expiration of that time, *if the officer be not able to travel*, he must make application to the Adjutant-General of the Army for an extension, accompanied by the certificate of a medical officer of the army, in the usual form, and that he is not able to travel. If it be not practicable to procure such a certificate, in consequence of there being no army physician in the place where the officer resides, the certificate of a citizen physician, *attested by a civil magistrate*, may be substituted.

All officers of the Regulars and Volunteers, except those on parole, now absent from duty with leave, will be considered "absent without leave" (*paragraph* 1326, *General Regulations*), unless they are found at their posts within fifteen days from the date of this order, or are authorized by orders from the Adjutant-General to be absent, which orders will in all cases be based on a certificate as above described, and must be exhibited to the paymaster before payment is made them.

All invalid and wounded officers who are able to travel, although their disability may not have been removed (*paragraph* 187, *General Regulations*), will repair, without delay—those from the East to Annapolis, to report to the General Commanding the Camp of Instruction; those from the West to report to the commanding officer of Camp Chase, Ohio. At those points they will remain until able to proceed to their regiments, or until an examining board may decide adversely on their ability to return to duty within a reasonable time, and orders may be given by the President for their discharge.

GENERAL ORDERS No. 63.

War Department, Adjutant-General's Office,
Washington, *June* 10, 1864.

APPOINTMENTS.—MEDICAL DEPARTMENT.

Assistant-Surgeon William A. Hammond, U. S. Army, to be Surgeon-General, with the rank of Brigadier-General, April 25, 1862, to fill an original vacancy.

William F. Okie, of Pennsylvania, to be Assistant-Surgeon, February 3, 1862, vice Herndon, dropped.

TO BE BRIGADE-SURGEONS.

Eugene F. Sanger, of Maine, November 10, 1861.
Robert K. Smith, of Pennsylvania, November 10 1861.

Frederick Seymour, of Ohio, December 24, 1861.
David P. Smith, of Massachusetts, December 24, 1861.
William C. Otterson, of New York, December 24, 1861.
John T. Hodgen, of Missouri, December 24, 1861.
Richard T. Wevill, of Pennsylvania, December 24, 1861
John B. G. Baxter, of Wisconsin, December 24, 1861.
Lavington Quick, of Pennsylvania, December 24, 1861.
Norman Gay, of Ohio, December 24, 1861.
George Rex, of Pennsylvania, December 24, 1861.
Rufus H. Johnson, of Ohio, December 24, 1861.
Thomas A. Worrall, of Pennsylvania, December 24, 1861.
Frank M. Hiester, of Pennsylvania, December 24, 1861.
Gaylord D. Beebe, of Illinois, December 24, 1861.
Meredith Clymer, of Pennsylvania, December 25, 1861.
Thomas W. Fry, of Missouri, January 17, 1862.
Edward E. Phelps, of Vermont, February 4, 1862.
Charles H. Rawson, of Iowa, February 19, 1862.
Alexander T. Watson, of New York, April 4, 1862.
J. H. Baxter, of Vermont, April 4, 1862.
W. H. Thorn, of Pennsylvania, April 4, 1862.
Bernard Beust, of New Jersey, April 4, 1862.
William W. Holmes, of Ohio, April 4, 1862.
E. Boyd Pendleton, of Virginia, April 4, 1862.
Samuel L. Bigelow, of France, April 4, 1862.
Jacob Bockee, of Illinois, April 4, 1862.
William W. Nassan, of Ohio, April 4, 1862.
William H. White, of Delaware, April 4, 1862.
Alfred Hitchcock, of Massachusetts, April 4, 1862.
Abraham Crispell, of New York, April 4, 1862.
Thomas B. Reed, of Pennsylvania, April 4, 1862.
Horace Wardner, of Illinois, April 4, 1862.
John B. Lewis, of Connecticut, April 4, 1862.
B. M. McVickar, of Illinois, April 4, 1862.
Frederick G. Snelling, of New York, April 4, 1862.
James C. Fisher, of New Jersey, April 4, 1862.
Edward D. Dailey, of Delaware, April 4, 1862.
J. T. Bradford, of Kentucky, April 4, 1862.
Azariah B. Shipman, of New York, April 4, 1862.
James G. Hatchitt, of Kentucky, April 4, 1862.
Abraham L. Cox, of New Jersey, April 4, 1862.
Alonzo J. Phelps, of Ohio, April 4, 1862.
Samuel M. Hamilton, of Illinois, April 4, 1862.
George T. Allen, of Illinois, April 4, 1862.
Augustus C. Hamlin, of Maine, April 4, 1862.
William Dickinson, of Missouri, April 4, 1862.
Ira Russell, of Massachusetts, April 4, 1862.
Isaac I. Hayes, of Pennsylvania, April 4, 1862.
Henry Palmer, of Wisconsin, April 4, 1862.
Ferris Jacobs, of New York April 4, 1862.

Clark McDermont, of Ohio, April 14, 1862.
Stephen F. Elliott, of California, April 21, 1862.
Daniel Holmes, of Pennsylvania, April 28, 1862.
George M. Kellogg, of Iowa, April 28, 1862.
Artemas Chapel, of Nebraska, May 1, 1862.
J. Theodore Heard, of Massachusetts, May 1, 1862.
John W. Hunt, of New York, May 12, 1862.

RETIRED.

Surgeon-General Clement A. Finley, U. S. Army, April 14, 1862, on his own application, after more than forty consecutive years of service.

DIED.

Surgeon Nathan Jarvis, at Baltimore, Maryland, May 12, 1862.

RESIGNED.

Brigade-Surgeon J. H. Warren, May 22, 1862.
Brigade-Surgeon Gilman Kimball, May 21, 1862.
Brigade-Surgeon Tarrant A. Perkins, March 24, 1862.
Brigade-Surgeon E. Boyd Pendleton, June 10, 1862.
Brigade-Surgeon B. McVickar, May 14, 1862.

APPOINTMENT NEGATIVED BY THE SENATE.

William Brodie as Brigade-Surgeon, February 3, 1862.

DECLINED.

By Joseph K. Van Pelt, of Pennsylvania, the appointment of Brigade-Surgeon.

By John T. B. McMaster, of Maryland, the appointment of Brigade-Surgeon.

DIED.

Brigade-Surgeon Luther V. Bell, at Camp on the Potomac River, Maryland, February 11, 1862.

DISMISSED.

Brigade-Surgeon J. H. Thompson, April 18, 1862.

DROPPED.

Assistant-Surgeon John J. Butler, May 17,1862.

GENERAL ORDERS No. 65.

War Department, Adjutant-General's Office,
Washington, *June* 12, 1862.

I. Paragraph 1269, Army Regulations, is hereby so modified, that Private Physicians, employed as Medical Officers with an Army in the field in time of war, may be allowed a sum not to exceed one hundred and twenty-five dollars per month, besides transportation in kind.

II. The certificates of discharge to be given by the Medical Inspector-General, or any Medical Inspector of the Army, under the Act of May 14, 1862, published in "General Orders," No. 53, will be made on the printed forms for Certificates of Disability, prescribed by the Army Regulations. The Inspector giving the discharge will endorse it with his own certificate that it is granted upon his own personal inspection of the soldier, and with the soldier's consent; and for disability, the nature, degree, and origin of which are correctly described in the within certificate.

III. Each Medical Director must, under the orders of his Department Commander, regulate the distribution of the sick and wounded to the hospitals within the Military Department to which he belongs. When want of room in such hospitals, or the nature of the wounds or disease of any invalids, require that detachments shall be sent beyond the limits of their departments, the Surgeon-General will designate to the Medical Directors, either by general instructions or specially by telegraph, to what points they shall be sent. Officers whose duty it may become to forward such detachments, will take care that no men, except those provided with written passes from their hospital surgeon or the Medical Director, shall be allowed to go.

Convalescents in Army Hospitals will be reported by the surgeons in charge to the Military Commanders, to be sent to camps or depôts, until they can be sent to join their regiments. Muster-rolls of each detachment will be made out from the best data at hand, the statement of the men being taken in the absence of other data concerning them. A duplicate of each muster-roll must be sent to the Adjutant-General the day the detachment starts.

GENERAL ORDERS No. 67.

War Department, Adjutant-General's Office,
Washington, *June* 17, 1862.

* * * Colonel William Hoffman, Third Infantry, Commissary-General of Prisoners, * * * will direct the manner in which all funds arising from the saving of rations at prison hospitals * * * shall be accounted for and disbursed. * * * * *

GENERAL ORDERS No. 68.

War Department, Adjutant-General's Office,
Washington, June 18, 1862.

1. Whenever soldiers are discharged while absent from their commands, the officers granting the discharge will furnish them with final statements for pay and certificates of discharge. The same officers, including Medical Inspectors, will in all cases notify the Adjutant-General and the Commanding Officer of the company to which the soldier belongs, of the date, place, and cause of such discharge. Certificates of disability are never to be given into the hands of the soldier, but will be forwarded to the Adjutant-General after being completed. (See paragraphs 167 and 168, General Regulations.)

GENERAL ORDERS No. 73.

War Department, Adjutant-General's Office,
Washington, *July* 4, 1862.

Promotions and Appointments in the Army of the United States, made by the President, by and with the Advice and Consent of the Senate, since the Publication of "General Orders No. 63, *of June* 10, 1862."

I. PROMOTIONS.—MEDICAL DEPARTMENT.

Assistant-Surgeon Jonathan Letterman, to be Surgeon, April 16, 1862, to fill an original vacancy.

Assistant-Surgeon Robert O. Abbott, to be Surgeon, April 16, 1862, to fill an original vacancy.

Assistant-Surgeon Thomas M. Getty, to be Surgeon, April 16, 1862, to fill an original vacancy.

Assistant-Surgeon David L. Magruder, to be Surgeon, April 16, 1862, to fill an original vacancy.

Assistant-Surgeon William J. H. White, to be Surgeon, April 16, 1862, to fill an original vacancy.

Assistant-Surgeon John J. Milhau, to be Surgeon, April 16, 1862, to fill an original vacancy.

Assistant-Surgeon Horace R. Wirtz, to be Surgeon, April 16, 1862, to fill an original vacancy.

Assistant-Surgeon Charles Page, to be Surgeon, April 16, 1862, to fill an original vacancy.

Assistant-Surgeon Charles Sutherland, to be Surgeon, April 16, 1862, to fill an original vacancy.

Assistant-Surgeon Basil Norris, to be Surgeon, April 16, 1862, to fill an original vacancy.

II. APPOINTMENTS.—MEDICAL DEPARTMENT.

Surgeon Robert C. Wood, to be Assistant Surgeon-General, with the rank of Colonel, June 14, 1862, to fill an original vacancy.

Brigade-Surgeon Thomas F. Perley, to be Medical Inspector-General, with the rank of Colonel, July 1, 1862, to fill an original vacancy.

Surgeon John M. Cuyler, to be Medical Inspector, with the rank of Lieutenant-Colonel, June 11, 1862, to fill an original vacancy.

Surgeon Richard H. Coolidge, to be Medical Inspector, with the rank of Lieutenant-Colonel, June 11, 1862, to fill an original vacancy.

Surgeon Charles C. Keeney, to be Medical Inspector, with the rank of Lieutenant-Colonel, June 11, 1862, to fill an original vacancy.

Assistant-Surgeon Edward P. Vollum, to be Medical Inspector, with the rank of Lieutenant-Colonel, June 11, 1862, to fill an original vacancy.

Brigade-Surgeon George H. Lyman, to be Medical Inspector, with the rank of Lieutenant-Colonel, June 11, 1862, to fill an original vacancy.

Brigade-Surgeon William H. Mussey, to be Medical Inspector, with the rank of Lieutenant-Colonel, June 14, 1862, to fill an original vacancy.

Brigade-Surgeon George T. Allen, to be Medical Inspector, with the rank of Lieutenant-Colonel, June 14, 1862, to fill an original vacancy.

Surgeon Lewis Humphreys, of the Twenty-ninth Regiment of Indiana Volunteers, to be Medical Inspector, with the rank of Lieutenant-Colonel, June 30, 1862, to fill an original vacancy.

John S. Billings, of Ohio, to be Assistant-Surgeon, April 16, 1862, *vice* Letterman, promoted.

Samuel Adams, of Maryland, to be Assistant-Surgeon, April 16, 1862, *vice* Abbott, promoted.

Edward T. Wittingham, of New Jersey, to be Assistant-Surgeon, April 16, 1862, *vice* Getty, promoted.

Phineas S. Conner, of Ohio, to be Assistant-Surgeon, April 16, 1862, *vice* Magruder, promoted.

Thomas G. Mackenzie, of Maryland, to be Assistant-Surgeon, April 16, 1862, *vice* White, promoted.

William I. Wolfley, of Kentucky, to be Assistant-Surgeon, April 16, 1862, *vice* Milhau, promoted.

William N. Notson, of Pennsylvania, to be Assistant-Surgeon, April 16, 1862, *vice* Wirtz, promoted.

John T. Riley, of Nebraska, to be Assistant-Surgeon, April 16, 1862, *vice* Page, promoted.

Edward de W. Breneman, of Pennsylvania, to be Assistant-Surgeon, April 16, 1862, *vice* Sutherland, promoted.

George M. McGill, of Pennsylvania, to be Assistant-Surgeon, April 16, 1862, *vice* Norris, promoted.

Jeremiah B. Brinton, of Pennsylvania, to be Assistant-Surgeon, April 16, 1862, to fill an original vacancy.

William E. Waters, of the District of Columbia, to be Assistant-Surgeon, April 16, 1862, to fill an original vacancy.

Robert B. Cruice, of Pennsylvania, to be Assistant-Surgeon, April 16, 1862, to fill an original vacancy.

Joseph R. Gibson, of Pennsylvania, to be Assistant-Surgeon, April 16, 1862, to fill an original vacancy.

Cyrus Bacon, Jr., of Michigan, to be Assistant-Surgeon, April 16, 1862, to fill an original vacancy.

S. H. Horner, of Pennsylvania, to be Assistant-Surgeon, April 16, 1862, to fill an original vacancy.

MEDICAL DEPARTMENT.—TO BE BRIGADE-SURGEONS.

Thomas B. Catlin, of New York, April 4, 1862.
Daniel W. Wainwright, of New York, June 9, 1862.
Aaron P. Dalrymple, of New York, June 9, 1862.
John L. LeConte, of Pennsylvania, June 9, 1862.
Burkitt Cloak, of Kentucky, June 9, 1862.
James C. Dorr, of Massachusetts, June 11, 1862.

Adam Hammer, of Missouri, June 14, 1862.
Edward McDonnell, of New York, June 21, 1862.
Charles L. Allen, of Vermont, June 23, 1862.
Henry Buckmaster, of Kansas, June 28, 1862.

DROPPED. (1.)

Assistant-Surgeon James C. Herndon, November 27, 1861.

COMMISSION VACATED BY NEW APPOINTMENT. (1.)

By Medical Inspector George H. Lyman, his commission as Brigade-Surgeon of Volunteers, June 24, 1862.

DECLINED. (1.)

By Alfred Hitchcock, of Massachusetts, the appointment of Brigade-Surgeon of Volunteers, April 4, 1862.

GENERAL ORDERS NO. 77.

War Department, Adjutant-General's Office,
Washington, *July* 11, 1862.

The following Act of Congress is published for the information of all concerned:

AN ACT making Appropriations for the Support of the Army for the Year ending the Thirtieth of June, Eighteen Hundred and Sixty-three, and additional Appropriations for the Year ending Thirtieth of June, Eighteen Hundred and Sixty-two, and for other Purposes.

Be it enacted by the Senate and House of Representatives of the United States of America in Congress assembled, That the following sums be, and the same are hereby appropriated, out of any money in the Treasury not otherwise appropriated, for the support of the army for the year ending the thirtieth of June, eighteen hundred and sixty-three.

For the recruiting service of the army, namely: For compensation to citizen-surgeons for medical attendance—one hundred and eighty thousand dollars.

For the medical and hospital department, including pay of private physicians, purchase and repair of surgical instruments, purchase of extra hospital bedding, clothing, ice, pay of male citizens as hospital attendants; the maintenance of sick and wounded soldiers placed in private houses or hospitals, and other necessary comforts for the sick and convalescing in the various military hospitals—five millions seven hundred and five thousand nine hundred and eighty-four dollars.

For pay of private physicians, purchase and repair of surgical instruments, purchase of extra hospital bedding, clothing, ice, and other necessary comforts for the sick and convalescing in the various military hospitals—one hundred and twenty-five thousand dollars.

For compensation of chaplains of hospitals, from the date of the commencement of their service to the thirtieth of June, eighteen hundred and sixty-two—twelve thousand dollars.

SEC. 10. *And be it further enacted*, That the Secretary of War be authorized to commute the army ration of coffee and sugar, for the extract of coffee, combined with milk and sugar, to be procured in the same manner and under like restrictions and guarantees as preserved meats, pickles, butter, and desiccated vegetables are procured for the navy, if he shall believe it will be conducive to the health and comfort of the army, and not more expensive to the Government than the present ration, and if it shall be acceptable to the men.

GENERAL ORDERS NO. 78.

War Department, Adjutant-General's Office,
Washington, *July* 14, 1862.

1. The many evils which arise from giving furloughs to enlisted men, require that the practice shall be discontinued. Hospitals provided with ample medical attendance, nurses, food, and clothing, are established by the Government, at great expense, not only near the scenes of active military operations but in many of the Northern States. When it is expedient and advisable, sick and wounded patients may, under the direction of the Surgeon-General, be transferred in parties, but not in individual cases; to hospitals at the North; and, as far as practicable, the men will be sent to States in which their regiments were raised, provided United States hospitals have been established there. Such regulations will be adopted at all the hospitals as will permit relatives and friends to visit the patients, and furnish them with comforts at such hour and in such manner as will not interfere with the discipline of the hospitals and the welfare of the mass of patients. The men will thus be under the fostering care of the Government while unfit for duty; will be in position to be promptly discharged, if proper, and, being always under military control, will be returned to their regiments as soon as able to resume their duties. The unauthorized removal of soldiers from under control of the United States authorities, by any agents whatever, subjects them to loss of pay and other penalties of desertion.

3. Chaplains appointed by the President for hospitals, will be assigned by the Surgeon-General to hospitals in cities for which they were appointed. Should the breaking up of a hospital leave a chaplain supernumerary in any city, the fact will be immediately reported to the Adjutant-General. Chaplains will be subordinate to the Hospital Surgeon. Leaves of absence will be granted them by the Surgeon-General, when approved by the surgeons in charge of their hospitals.

GENERAL ORDERS No. 85.

War Department, Adjutant-General's Office,
Washington, *July* 23, 1862.

The following order is published for the information of the Army :

War Department, Washington City, D. C., *July* 22, 1862.

Order in Respect to Clothing for Sick and Wounded Soldiers.

The following is a Joint Resolution of Congress, approved 12th July, 1862:

JOINT RESOLUTION authorizing the Secretary of War to Furnish Extra Clothing to Sick, Wounded, and other Soldiers.

Resolved by the Senate and House of Representatives of the United States of America in Congress assembled, That the Secretary of War be authorized to furnish extra clothing to all sick, wounded, and other soldiers who may have lost the same by casualties of war, under such rules and regulations as the Department may prescribe, during the existence of the present rebellion.

In pursuance of the foregoing resolution, it is ordered, That the Quartermaster's Department shall issue, upon the requisition of the Medical Officer in charge of any hospital or depôt of sick and wounded soldiers, such regulation clothing, necessary to their health and comfort, as may be requisite to replace that lost by them from the casualties of the war. The necessity of the issue to be certified by the Surgeon, and the requisition to be approved by the Medical Director or Medical Inspector of the station. Such issue to be gratuitous and not charged to the soldier.

The Quartermaster-General will cause blank requisitions to be furnished to the officers of the various hospitals upon their application.

GENERAL ORDERS No. 86.

War Department, Adjutant-General's Office,
Washington, *July* 23, 1862.

I. *Descriptive lists* and *accounts* of the *pay*, *clothing*, &c., of soldiers, will never, where it can be avoided, be given into their own hands. Such papers should be intrusted only to the officer or non-commissioned officer in charge of the party with which they are.

II. Except in such cases as that of an Ordnance Sergeant, specially assigned to duty at a post where there are no troops, and where he cannot be regularly mustered, *no soldier must be paid on a mere descriptive list and account of pay and clothing*, but only upon the muster and pay-roll of his company, detachment, or party, or on that of a general hospital, if he be there sick or on duty. *No payments will, therefore, be made to enlisted men on furlough.*

III. The giving *in duplicate*, by any officer of the army, of *certificates of discharge*, or *final statements*, is peremptorily forbidden (see paragraph 165 of the Revised Regulations). Not even if such papers are lost or destroyed, is any officer of the army authorized to replace them.

IV. The proper course to be pursued in such cases will be found indicated in paragraph 1341 of the Revised Regulations, and is substantially as follows:

Application for payment in these cases must be made *through the Paymaster-General of the Army*, to the Second Comptroller of the Treasury. The application must be accompanied by the soldier's statement, under oath, that his final statements and certificate of discharge are lost, destroyed, or have never been received by him; that he has made diligent search or application for them; that they cannot be recovered or obtained; and that he has not received pay on them, nor assigned them to any other person.

All the circumstances of the case must be fully set forth in the affidavit, and this again must be accompanied by all the evidence in corroboration of his statement, which the soldier can procure.

On receipt of this, the Second Comptroller will audit the account, and, if satisfied with the evidence, will order payment to the soldier of the amount found justly due to him.

GENERAL ORDERS No. 87.

War Department, Adjutant-General's Office,
Washington, *July* 24, 1862.

Promotions and Appointments in the Army of the United States, made by the President, by and with the Advice and Consent of the Senate, since the Publication of " General Orders," No. 73, *of July* 4, 1862.

MEDICAL DEPARTMENT.—PROMOTIONS.

Assistant-Surgeon John Moore, to be Surgeon, May 12, 1862, *vice* Jarvis, deceased.

Assistant-Surgeon Andrew K. Smith, to be Surgeon, June 11, 1862, *vice* Cuyler, appointed Medical Inspector.

Assistant-Surgeon Richard H. Alexander, to be Surgeon, June 11, 1862, *vice* Coolidge, appointed Medical Inspector.

Assistant-Surgeon Joseph R. Smith, to be Surgeon, June 11, 1862, *vice* Keeney, appointed Medical Inspector.

MEDICAL DEPARTMENT.—APPOINTMENTS.

William W. Keen, of Pennsylvania, to be Assistant-Surgeon, July 11, 1862, to fill an original vacancy.

George L. Porter, of Pennsylvania, to be Assistant-Surgeon, July 11, 1862, to fill an original vacancy.

David L. Huntingdon, of Pennsylvania, to be Assistant-Surgeon, July 11, 1862, to fill an original vacancy.

T. W. Williams, of the District of Columbia, to be Assistant-Surgeon, July 11, 1862, to fill an original vacancy.

Charles M. Colton, of Virginia, to be Assistant-Surgeon, July 11, 1862, *vice* Hammond, appointed Surgeon-General.

T. M. Brown, of Ohio, to be Assistant-Surgeon, July 11, 1862, *vice* Moore, promoted.

Charles S. De Graw, of New York, to be Assistant-Surgeon, July 11, 1861, *vice* A. K. Smith, promoted.

Edward C. Strode, of Illinois, to be Assistant-Surgeon, July 11, 1862, *vice* Vollum, appointed Medical Inspector.

Andrew H. Smith, of New York, to be Assistant-Surgeon, July 11, 1862, *vice* Alexander, promoted.

Van Buren Hubbard, of Ohio, to be Assistant-Surgeon, July 11, 1862, *vice* J. R. Smith, promoted.

GENERAL ORDERS No. 90.

War Department, Adjutant-General's Office,
Washington, *July* 26, 1862.

I. The principle being recognised that Chaplains should not be held as prisoners of war, it is hereby ordered that all Chaplains so held by the United States shall be immediately and unconditionally discharged.

GENERAL ORDERS No. 91.

War Department, Adjutant-General's Office,
Washington, *July* 29, 1862.

The following Acts of Congress are published for the information of all concerned.

AN ACT to define the Pay and Emoluments of Certain Officers of the Army and for other Purposes.

Sect. 8. *And be it further enacted*, That so much of section nine of the aforesaid act, approved July 22, 1861, and of section seven of the "Act providing for the better Organization of the Military Establishment," approved August 3, 1861, as defines the qualifications of Chaplains in the Army and Volunteers, shall be hereafter construed to read as follows: That no person shall be appointed a Chaplain in the United States Army, who is not a regularly ordained minister of some religious denomination, and who does not present testimonials of his present good standing as such minister, from some ecclesiastical body or not less than five accredited ministers belonging to said religious denomination.

Section 9. *And be it further enacted*, That hereafter the compensation of all Chaplains in the Regular or Volunteer service, or Army Hospitals, shall be one hundred dollars per month, and two rations per day when on duty. * * Chaplains employed at the military posts called "Chaplain posts," shall be required to reside at the posts, and all Chaplains in the United States service shall be subject to such rules in relation to leave of absence from duty as are prescribed for commissioned officers of the United States Army, stationed at such posts.

Sect. 11. *And be it further enacted*, That the cavalry forces in the service of the United States shall hereafter be organized as follows: Each regiment of cavalry shall have * * * one Surgeon, one Assistant-Surgeon, two Hospital Stewards. * *

GENERAL ORDERS NO. 126.

War Department, Adjutant-General's Office,
Washington, *September* 6, 1862.

1. The following is the organization of regiments and companies of the volunteer army of the United States:

REGIMENT OF INFANTRY.

1 Surgeon; 2 Assistant-Surgeons; 1 Hospital Steward.

REGIMENT OF CAVALRY.

1 Surgeon; 1 Assistant-Surgeon; 2 Hospital Stewards.

REGIMENT OF ARTILLERY.

1 Hospital Steward.

GENERAL ORDERS NO. 131.

War Department, Adjutant-General's Office,
Washington, *September* 16, 1862.

By direction of the President the following officers are dismissed from the service:

Surgeon Lyman H. Stone, U.S.A. * * * *

GENERAL ORDERS NO. 132.

War Department, Adjutant-General's Office,
Washington, *September* 17, 1862.

Ordered, That Medical Purveyors be required to give bond in the sum of seventy-five thousand dollars.

GENERAL ORDERS NO. 160.

War Department, Adjutant-General's Office,
Washington, *October* 18, 1862.

The following regulations are established for Army Trains and Baggage:

II. The wagons allowed to a regiment, battery, or squadron, must carry nothing but forage for the teams, cooking utensils, and rations for the troops, hospital stores, and officers' baggage. *One wagon to each regiment will transport exclusively hospital supplies, under the direction of the Regimental Surgeon;* the one for regimental headquarters will carry the grain for the officers' horses; and the three allowed for each battery or squadron, will be at least half loaded with grain for their own teams.

V. Hospital tents are for the sick and wounded, and, except those allowed for Army Corps Headquarters, must not be diverted from their proper use.

GENERAL ORDERS NO. 179.

War Department, Adjutant-General's Office,
Washington, *October* 31, 1862.

Paragraph 1 of "General Orders," No. 92, of October 26, 1861, is so far modified as to require the submission to the Secretary of

War of plans for hospital accommodation of the sick, only in cases which, in the opinion of the Quartermaster General, or of the Surgeon-General, require special action of the Secretary.

GENERAL ORDERS NO. 177.

War Department, Adjutant-General's Office,
Washington, *October* 31, 1862.

The regiments and companies of Volunteer Engineers, recognised by the 20th section of the Act of July 17, 1862, will have the following organization:

REGIMENT OF ENGINEERS—TWELVE COMPANIES.

1 Chaplain; 1 Surgeon; 2 Assistant-Surgeons; 1 Hospital Steward.

GENERAL ORDERS NO. 181.

War Department, Adjutant-General's Office,
Washington, *November* 1, 1862.

I. MEDICAL DEPARTMENT.—PROMOTIONS.

Assist.-Surgeon George Taylor, to be Surgeon, August 27, 1862, *vice* Porter, retired.

Asst.-Surgeon B. J. D. Irwin, to be Surgeon, September 16, 1862, *vice* Stone, dismissed.

II. APPOINTMENTS.

Harrison Allen, of Pennsylvania, to be Assistant-Surgeon, July 30, 1862.

William P. Grier, of Pennsylvania, to be Assistant-Surgeon, July 30, 1862.

Thomas McMillan, of Kentucky, to be Assistant-Surgeon, August 12, 1862.

Edward Brooks, of New York, to be Assistant-Surgeon, August 19, 1862.

Charles P. Russell, of New York, to be Assistant-Surgeon, September 4, 1862.

Thomas H. Ridgely, of Pennsylvania, to be Assistant-Surgeon, September 16, 1862.

MEDICAL STOREKEEPERS.

Hennel Stevens, of Connecticut, August 13, 1862.
Henry N. Rittenhouse, of Pennsylvania, August 13, 1862.
Victor Zoeller, of New York, August 13, 1862.
Henry Johnson, of Pennsylvania, August 13, 1862.
Robert T. Creamer, of New York, August 13, 1862.
Hospital Steward George Wright, U.S.A., August 13, 1862.

TO BE SURGEONS OF VOLUNTEERS, AUGUST 8, 1862.

Morse K. Taylor, of Illinois.
Francis Bacon, of Connecticut.
Thomas McMartin, of Missouri.

SEPTEMBER 11, 1862.

Alfred Wynkoop, of Pennsylvania.
R. Cresson Stiles, of Massachusetts.
Thomas R. Crosby, of New Hampshire.

SEPTEMBER 12, 1862.

Edward Shippen, of Pennsylvania.
Zenas E. Bliss, of Michigan.

OCTOBER 4, 1864.

Henry S. Churchman, of Illinois.
Paul B. Goddard, of Pennsylvania.
Hayes Agnew, of Pennsylvania.
Alpheus B. Crosby, of New Hampshire.
Joseph Hopkinson, of Pennsylvania.
Henry A. Martin, of Massachusetts.
John R McClurg, of Pennsylvania.
Barton Darrach, of Illinois.
Clayton A. Cowgill, of Delaware.
Bowman B. Breed, of Massachusetts.
Sylvanus D. Freeman, of Pennsylvania.
Israel Moses, of New York.

ASSISTANT-SURGEONS OF VOLUNTEERS.

Calvin G. Page, of Massachusetts, August 8, 1862.

SEPTEMBER 11, 1862.

Augustus M. Clark, of New York.
F. Townsend Dade, of Pennsylvania.
James H. Wythes, of Pennsylvania.
James Phillips, of ——
Elmore Y. Chase, of Ohio
John M. Robinson, of ——.
Conrad C. Dumreicher, of Illinois.
David B. Sturgeon, of Pennsylvania.
Geo. W. Hogeboom, of Missouri.
William S. Thompson, of Pennsylvania.
John Wilson, of Pennsylvania.
Andrew B. Chapin, of Michigan.

OCTOBER 4, 1862.

William Moss, of Pennsylvania.
John W. Brewer, of Maryland.
George L. Sutton, of New York.
Andrew F. Sheldon, of New York.
George A. Pattee, of Canada.
William A. Conover, of New Jersey.
Peter Cleary, of New York.

Edward Dodd, of New York.
Charles S. Frink, of Indiana.
George A. Wheeler, of Maine.
Sylvanus S. Mulford, of New York.
Frederick A. Keffer, of Pennsylvania.
Adolf Majer, of New York.
Henry Parker, of Massachusetts.
Augustus C. Van Duyn, of New York.

RETIRED.

Surgeon Samuel G. I. De Camp, August 27, 1862, from incapacity resulting from long and faithful service, and of sickness consequent to exposure in the line of his duty.

Surgeon John B. Porter, Surgeon William F. Edgar, and Assistant-Surgeon Joseph H. Bailey, same date and for same cause as stated in case of Surgeon De Camp.

RESIGNED.

Assist.-Surgeon Richard D. Lynde, August 31, 1862.
Assist.-Surgeon Josiah F. Kennedy, October 10, 1862.
Hospital Chaplain Isaac O. Sloan, September 9, 1862.
Hospital Chaplain Albert Paine, August 28, 1862.
Hospital Chaplain O. S. Prescott, September 29, 1862.
Surgeon S. L. Herrick, August 17, 1862.
Surgeon Chas. H. Rawson, August 22, 1862.
Surgeon Daniel McRuer, September 2, 1862.
Surgeon Daniel Holmes, September 10, 1862.
Surgeon W. C. Thompson, September 19, 1862.
Surgeon David Prince, September 22, 1862.
Surgeon Robert Roskoton, July 25, 1862.
Surgeon George C. Blackman, July 31, 1862.
Assist.-Surgeon Calvin G. Page, August 28, 1862.

DECLINED.

By William J. Wolfley, of Kentucky, and William W. Keen, of Pennsylvania, the appointment of Assistant-Surgeon, U. S. Army.

By H. A. Buck of Illinois, A. McMahon of Ohio, and B. S. Forbes of Pennsylvania, the appointment of Assistant-Surgeon of Volunteers.

DIED.

Surgeon William J. H. White, killed at the battle of Antietam Md., September 17, 1862.

GENERAL ORDERS NO. 8.

War Department, Adjutant-General's Office,
Washington, *January* 3, 1863.

The following Act of Congress is published for the information and government of all concerned:

AN ACT to facilitate the Discharge of Disabled Soldiers from the Army, and the Inspection of Convalescent Camps and Hospitals.

[PUBLIC—No. 5.]

Be it enacted by the Senate and House of Representatives of the United States of America in Congress assembled, That there shall be added to the present medical corps of the army eight Medical Inspectors, who shall, immediately after the passage of this Act, be appointed by the President, by and with the advice and consent of the Senate, without regard to their rank when so selected, but with sole regard to qualifications, and who shall have the rank, pay, and emoluments now authorized by law to officers of that grade.

SEC. 2. *And be it further enacted,* That the officers of the Medical Inspector's department shall be charged, in addition to the duties now assigned to them by existing laws, with the duty of making regular and frequent inspections of all military general hospitals and convalescent camps, and shall, upon each such inspection, designate to the surgeon in charge of such hospitals or camps all soldiers who may be, in their opinion, fit subjects for discharge from the service, on surgeon's certificate of disability, or sufficiently recovered to be returned to their regiments for duty, and shall see that such soldiers are discharged or so returned. And the Medical inspecting officers are hereby empowered, under such regulations as may be hereafter established, to direct the return to duty, or the discharge from service, as the case may be, of all soldiers designated by them.

Approved December 27, 1862.

GENERAL ORDERS NO. 4.

War Department, Adjutant-General's Office,
Washington, *January* 5, 1863.

I. By direction of the President, Assistant-Surgeon G. E. Pattee, U. S. Volunteers, is dropped from the rolls of the army, for absence without leave, to take effect October 14, 1862.

GENERAL ORDERS NO. 15.

War Department, Adjutant-General's Office,
Washington, *January* 19, 1863.

I. Assistant-Surgeon A. J. Baxter, U. S. Army, is, by direction of the President, hereby dismissed the service of the United States.

GENERAL ORDERS NO. 19

War Department, Adjutant-General's Office,
Washington, *January* 23, 1863.

I. By direction of the President, Hospital Chaplain C. W. Denison, having left this country for Europe, is dropped from the rolls of the Army.

II. By direction of the President, Surgeon William W. Nassau,* U. S. Volunteers, is dismissed the service of the United States.

---

* Revoked.

GENERAL ORDERS NO. 30.

War Department, Adjutant-General's Office,
Washington, *February* 4, 1863.

Paragraph 1341, General Regulations, and "General Orders," No. 86, of July 23, 1862, paragraph IV., are hereby modified so as to require that applications for payment in cases where certificates of discharge or final statements are lost or destroyed, shall be made to the Second Auditor of the Treasury instead of the Second Comptroller.

CIRCULAR NO. 16.

War Department, Adjutant-General's Office,
Washington, *February* 6, 1864.

In future, each officer in charge of enlisted men absent from their regiments will report at the end of every month to the Regimental or Company Commanders of the men under their charge, whether they are sick, in confinement, in hospital, or detached service, &c.; their station, the duties which each man is performing, and the authority for detaining him, giving the number and date of the order. Also whether they are sick, or fit for service, and any other particulars about them which may be necessary for the information of their commanding officers in keeping a correct account of the pay, clothing, station, duties, &c., of each soldier. Without such reports, men cannot receive the pay actually due them.

GENERAL ORDERS NO. 39.

War Department, Adjutant-General's Office,
Washington, *February* 10, 1863.

II. Surgeons George S. Kemble* and Thomas McMartin, U. S. Volunteers, are, by direction of the President, honorably discharged the service of the United States on account of ill health.

GENERAL ORDERS NO. 40.

War Department, Adjutant-General's Office,
Washington, *February* 11, 1863.

The following Acts of Congress are published for the information and government of all concerned:

An Act making Appropriations for the Support of the Army for the year ending the Thirtieth of June, Eighteen Hundred and Sixty-four, and for a deficiency for the Signal Service for the Year ending June Thirty, Eighteen Hundred and Sixty-three.

For medicines, instruments, dressings, and so forth, for the regular army, one hundred and fifty-five thousand dollars.

For hospital stores, bedding, and so forth, for the regular army, one hundred thousand dollars.

For hospital furniture and field equipments, for the regular army, thirty thousand dollars.

---

* Restored.

For medical books, stationery, and printing, for the regular army, eight thousand seven hundred and fifty dollars.

For private physicians and medicines furnished by them, for the regular army, fifty-seven thousand five hundred dollars.

For hire of clerks and laborers in purveying depôts, for the regular army, one thousand six hundred dollars.

For continuing meteorological observations and tabulating the same, under the direction of the Surgeon-General, for the regular army, five hundred dollars.

For contingencies, for the regular army, two thousand one hundred and fifty dollars.

For compensation of soldiers acting as cooks and nurses, under the acts of August sixteen, eighteen hundred and fifty-six, and March three, eighteen hundred and fifty-seven, for the regular army, two thousand dollars.

For ice, fruits, and other comforts, under acts of August three, eighteen hundred and sixty-one, and July five, eighteen hundred and sixty-two, for the regular army, twenty thousand dollars.

For citizen-nurses, under act of July five, eighteen hundred and sixty-two, for the regular army, four thousand dollars.

For hospital clothing for the regular army, fifteen thousand dollars.

For care of sick soldiers in private hospitals, for the regular army, eighteen thousand five hundred dollars.

For artificial limbs for soldiers, for the regular army, and seamen, five thousand dollars.

For medicines, instruments, dressings, and so forth, for the volunteers, four millions of dollars.

For hospital stores, bedding, and so forth, for the volunteers, three million five hundred thousand dollars.

For hospital furniture and field equipments, for the volunteers, one million dollars.

For medical books, stationery, and printing, for the volunteers, one hundred thousand dollars.

For private physicians and medicines furnished by them for the volunteers, four hundred thousand dollars.

For hire of clerks and laborers in purveying depôts for the volunteers, twenty-five thousand dollars.

For continuing meteorological observations and tabulating the same, under the direction of the Surgeon-General, for the volunteers, one thousand dollars.

For contingencies for the volunteers, twelve thousand five hundred dollars.

For compensation of soldiers acting as cooks and nurses, under the acts of August sixteen, eighteen hundred and fifty-six, and March three, eighteen hundred and fifty-seven, for the volunteers, seventy-five thousand dollars.

For ice, fruits, and other comforts, under acts of August three, eighteen hundred and sixty-one, and July one, eighteen hundred and sixty-two, for the volunteers, one hundred and seventy thousand dollars.

For citizen nurses, under act of July five, eighteen hundred and sixty-two, for the volunteers, one hundred thousand dollars.

For hospital clothing, for the volunteers, eighty thousand dollars.

For care of sick soldiers in private hospitals, for the volunteers, one hundred and sixteen thousand five hundred dollars.

For artificial limbs for volunteers, soldiers, and seamen, forty-five thousand dollars.

For the army medical museum, five thousand dollars.

For medicines and medical attendance for negro refugees (commonly called contrabands), fifty thousand dollars.

GENERAL ORDERS NO. 69.

War Department, Adjutant-General's Office,
Washington, *March* 20, 1863.

Paragraph 10 of General Orders, No. 36, of 1862, which authorizes the chief medical officer in each city "to employ as cooks, nurses, and attendants any convalescent, wounded, or feeble men who can perform such duties, instead of giving them discharges," is hereby modified as follows:

At every U. S. General Hospital, the feeble and wounded men, unfit for field duty, but not entirely disabled, instead of being discharged, will be organized and mustered in detachments, under the charge of the officers acting as Military Commanders, who will assign men to them from time to time, on the reports of the surgeons in charge of hospitals. From these Invalid detachments the Military Commanders will make details for provost, hospital, and other necessary guards; for clerks, hospital attendants, nurses, cooks, and other "extra duty" men.

The Invalid Detachments will be mustered and reported as detachments, and will be paid on the Detachment Rolls; but no *extra* pay will be allowed in any case.

The Detachment Rolls must show to what company and regiment each man properly belongs, and all assignments to them must be promptly reported to their company commanders. They are not to be dropped from the rolls of those companies, but will be reported on detached service from them.

Should any of the men become fit for duty with their regiments, they will be immediately sent to join them.

In case of a want of non-commissioned officers to give efficiency to the Invalid Detachments, lance appointments may be made, but without increase of pay.

GENERAL ORDERS NO. 72.

War Department, Adjutant-General's Office,
Washington, *March* 24, 1863.

Commanders of regiments, battalions not included in regiments, independent companies or batteries, and detachments, surgeons in charge of hospitals or detachments, and all persons in the military service, commanding or controlling commissioned officers or enlisted men on special or detached service, will report upon the last day of each month to Colonel James B. Fry, Provost-Marshal-General of the United States, at Washington, D.C., the names of all deserters from their respective commands who have deserted since their last report, or who have not previously been reported. These reports will be made in the form of descriptive lists, setting forth, in case of each deserter, his name, rank, regiment or company, description, place of birth, residence, occupation, place of enlistment, date of last payment, amount of bounty due, date and place of desertion, and the place where he can probably be found, with such other remarks as may be pertinent in the matter, or may aid in the arrest and punishment of the offender. Where no desertions have taken place during the month, the regular form of descriptive list will be forwarded, and the fact will be noted upon it. The lists will in all cases be made in duplicate; one copy will be forwarded direct to the Provost-Marshal-General, and the other, through the ordinary military channels, to the Adjutant-General, at Washington, who will refer the same to the Provost-Marshal-General. When lists are rendered by surgeons, one copy will be sent direct to the Provost-Marshal-General, and the duplicate, through the regular channel, to the Surgeon-General, who will refer the same to the Provost-Marshal-General.

GENERAL ORDERS NO. 73.

War Department, Adjutant-General's Office,
Washington, *March* 24, 1863.

The following Acts and Resolutions of Congress are published for the information of all concerned:

A Resolution to facilitate the Payment of Sick and Wounded Soldiers in the Hospitals and Convalescent Camps.

Resolved by the Senate and House of Representatives of the United States of America in Congress assembled, That the Paymaster-General be, and he hereby is, authorized and directed to take immediate measures for the prompt payment of the sick and wounded soldiers in the convalescent camps, hospitals, and elsewhere, so that they may be fully paid within sixty days from and after the passage hereof.

Approved March 3, 1863.

An Act for the Relief of Certain Persons who have performed the Duties of Assistant-Surgeons in Regiments of Cavalry.

Be it enacted by the Senate and House of Representatives of the United States of America in Congress assembled, That Physicians and Surgeons who have since the second day of July last been duly appointed and commissioned as Second Assistant-Surgeons in Volunteer Regiments of Cavalry, and as such have been duly mustered into the military service of the United States, and actually performed the duties appertaining to that office, shall be paid therefor in like manner and upon like proof as other Assistant-Surgeons of

Cavalry: *Provided*, That not more than two Assistant-Surgeons to each regiment shall be allowed and paid for services performed at one and the same time.

Approved March 3, 1863.

GENERAL ORDERS NO. 80.

War Department, Adjutant-General's Office,
Washington, *March* 31, 1863.

It is hereby ordered that all Surgeons and Assistant-Surgeons belonging to regiments, who are absent on any other than regimental duty, shall without delay rejoin their regiments. Medical officers of regiments will not hereafter be detached upon other service, except temporarily in cases of necessity, or where the Surgeon and two Assistant-Surgeons are present, when one of the Assistants may be detached to hospital duty.

GENERAL ORDERS NO. 86.

War Department, Adjutant-General's Office,
Washington, *April* 2, 1863.

I. Under the authority contained in Sections 19 and 20 of the act "for enrolling and calling out the national forces, and for other purposes," approved March 3, 1863, it is ordered that for each and every regiment of the volunteer army *now reduced, or that may be reduced hereafter, as set forth in said sections*, consolidation shall be made in accordance with the following rules:

INFANTRY.

1. Each regiment will be consolidated into *five, or a less number of companies*, and the Colonel, Major, and one Assistant-Surgeon mustered out.

CAVALRY.

2. Each regiment will be consolidated into *six, or a less number of companies*, and the Colonel, two Majors, and one Assistant-Surgeon mustered out.

ARTILLERY.

3. Each regiment will be consolidated into *six, or a less number of batteries*, and the Colonel, two Majors, and one Assistant-Surgeon mustered out.

GENERAL ORDERS NO. 87.

War Department, Adjutant-General's Office,
Washington, *April* 3, 1863.

I. Transportation for sanitary supplies will be furnished only on the requisition of a Medical Director, and when sent to another Department, the supplies must be assigned to the Medical Director of that Department.

II. The Assistant Surgeon-General, Medical Inspector-General, and Medical Inspectors will be allowed the same number of rooms as offices, and fuel and furniture therefor, as are allowed by Regulations to officers of the Quartermaster's Department who perform similar duties.

GENERAL ORDERS NO. 122.

War Department, Adjutant-General's Office,
Washington, *May* 14, 1863.

General Orders, No. 48, of 1862, paragraph II., is modified as follows:

Transportation for private physicians and nurses to attend sick and wounded soldiers will be provided by the Quartermaster's Department, upon the special order of the General commanding a Military Department, or an army in the field.

GENERAL ORDERS NO. 130.

War Department, Adjutant-General's Office,
Washington, *May* 15, 1863.

In executing the provisions of General Orders, No. 105, from this Department, in regard to the selection of men for the Invalid Corps, Medical Inspectors, Surgeons in charge of Hospitals, Camps, Regiments, or of Boards of Enrolment, Military Commanders, and all others required to make the physical examination of men for the Invalid Corps, will be governed in their decisions by the following list of qualifications and disqualifications for admission into this Corps:

Physical Infirmities that do not disqualify Enlisted Men for Service in the "Invalid Corps."

1. Paralysis, if confined to the left upper extremity, and the man's previous occupation fit him for the duty of clerk, orderly, etc.
2. Simple hypertrophy of the heart unaccompanied by valvular lesion; functional derangement of the stomach (dyspepsia); mild chronic diarrhœa; simple enlargement of the liver or spleen; a temporary ailment of the kidneys or bladder.
3. Chronic rheumatism, unless manifested by positive change of structure, wasting of the affected limb, or puffiness or distortion of the joints.
4. Pain, unless accompanied with manifest derangement of the general health, wasting of a limb, or other positive sign of disease.
5. Myopia, unless very decided or depending upon structural change of the eye.
6. Stammering, unless excessive and confirmed.
7. Loss of teeth or unsound teeth.
8. Torticollis.
9. Reducible hernia.
10. Hæmorrhoids.
11. Stricture of the urethra.
12. Incontinence of urine.
13. Loss or complete atrophy of both testicles from any cause;

permanent retention of one or both testicles within the inguinal canal.

14. Varicocele and circocele.

15. Loss of left arm, left forearm, or left hand, if the man be qualified for duty of clerk or orderly.

16. Loss of leg or foot, provided the man have the inclination and aptitude for service in a General Hospital, and is recommended for that duty by a medical officer, or if qualified for the duty of clerk or orderly.

17. Old and irreducible dislocation of shoulder and elbow in which the bones have accommodated themselves to their new relations.

18. Muscular and cutaneous contraction of left arm, provided the man may be employed as clerk, orderly, or messenger.

19. Loss of left thumb; partial loss of either thumb.

20. Loss of first and second phalanges of all the fingers of the left hand.

21. Total loss of any two fingers of the same hand.

22. Total loss of index finger of right hand.

23. Permanent extension of any finger of the right hand; permanent extension or contraction of any finger of the left hand.

24. Adherent or united fingers.

25. Loss of any toe or toes except the great toe; all the toes joined together.

26. Deformities of the toes, if not sufficient to prevent walking.

27. Large, flat, ill-shaped feet that do not come within the designation of talipes valgus.

28. Varicose veins not accompanied with ulcerations.

29. Gunshot wounds or injuries not involving loss of function.

30. None of the foregoing infirmities disqualify officers for service in the Invalid Corps.

In all cases where the physical infirmities of officers or enlisted men come within the provisions of the above list, they will be recommended for transfer to, or enlistment in, the Invalid Corps; but no one will be admitted into this Corps, whose previous record does not show that he is meritorious and deserving, and that he has complied with the provisions of General Orders, No. 105, War Department, Adjutant-General's Office, 1863, authorizing an Invalid Corps.

Physical Infirmities that disqualify Enlisted Men for Service in the Invalid Corps.

1. Manifest imbecility or insanity.

2. Epilepsy, if the seizures occur more frequently than once a month, and have obviously impaired the mental faculties.

3. Paralysis or chorea.

4. Acute or organic diseases of the brain or spinal cord; of the heart or lungs; of the stomach or intestines; of the liver or spleen;

of the kidneys or bladder, sufficient to have impaired the general health, or so well marked as to leave no reasonable doubt of the man's incapacity for military service.

5. Confirmed consumption; cancer; aneurism of important arteries.

6. Inveterate and extensive disease of the skin.

7. Scrofula, or constitutional syphilis, which has resisted treatment and seriously impaired the general health.

8. Habitual or confirmed intemperance, or solitary vice, sufficient in degree to have materially enfeebled the constitution.

9. Great injuries or diseases of the skull, occasioning impairment of the intellectual faculties, epilepsy, or other serious nervous or spasmodic symptoms.

10. Total loss of sight, or other serious diseases of the eye, affecting its integrity or use.

11. Loss of nose, or deformity of nose, if sufficient seriously to obstruct respiration; ozœna, if dependent upon caries.

12. Deafness.

13. Dumbness; permanent loss of voice.

14. Total loss of tongue, partial loss, and hypertrophy or atrophy of tongue, if sufficient to make the speech unintelligible and prevent mastication or deglutition.

15. Incurable deformities of either jaw, whether congenital or produced by accident, which would prevent mastication or greatly injure the speech.

16. Tumors of the neck impeding respiration or deglutition; fistula of larynx or trachea.

17. Deformity of the chest, sufficient to impede respiration, or to prevent the carrying of arms and military equipments; caries of the ribs; gunshot wound of the lung, if complicated with fracture of a rib.

18. Artificial anus; severe stricture of the rectum.

19. Total loss, or nearly total loss, of penis; epispadia, or hypospadia, at the middle or nearer the root of penis; stone in the bladder.

20. Confirmed or malignant sarcocele; hydrocele, if complicated with organic disease of the testis.

21. Excessive anterior or posterior curvature of spine; caries of the spine; lumbar abscess.

22. Loss of a thigh.

23. Wounds, fractures, tumors, atrophy of a limb, or chronic diseases of the joints or bone that would prevent marching or any considerable muscular exertion.

24. Anchylosis, or irreducible dislocation of the shoulder, elbow, wrist, hip, knee, or ankle-joint.

25. Muscular or cutaneous contractions from wounds or burns in degree sufficient to prevent useful motion of the right arm or of the lower extremities.

26. With the exception of those paragraphs which refer to the total or partial loss of an extremity, the foregoing disabilities dis-

qualify officers as well as enlisted men for service in the Invalid Corps.

In all cases where the physical infirmities of an officer or enlisted man come within the provisions of this list, or where his previous record shows that he is not entitled to be received into the Invalid Corps, he will, if in service, be discharged, and if an applicant to re-enter, his application will be disapproved.

Whilst the Government is most anxious to provide for and employ, to the best of their abilities, those faithful soldiers who, from wounds or the hardships of war, are no longer able to perform active duty in the field, yet it can, upon no account, permit men, undeserving or totally disabled, to re-enter its service.

Those faithful soldiers whose physical infirmities are too great to admit of their being of any use in the Invalid Corps will, nevertheless, receive the pensions and bounties provided by law.

It is further announced that no officer or enlisted man shall be entitled to or receive any pension, premium, or bounty, for enlistment, re-enlistment, or service in the Invalid Corps. They will receive all other pay and allowances now authorized by law for the U. S. Infantry except the increased pay for re-enlistment. Claims for pensions or bounties which may be due for previous services will not be invalidated by enlistment in the Invalid Corps. But no pensions can be drawn or accrue to the benefit of any man during his service in said Corps. The officers and men will be organized into companies of Infantry, of the same strength as is now authorized by law for the U. S. Infantry. No organized Brigades, Regiments, Companies, or parts of Companies, will be accepted as such. Enlistments in this Corps will be for three years, unless sooner discharged.

GENERAL ORDERS NO. 137.

War Department, Adjutant-General's Office,
Washington, *May* 18, 1863.

I. Whenever enlisted men are discharged, after two years' service, under circumstances that entitle them to the bounty provided by the 6th section of the Act of Congress approved July 22, and the 5th section of the Act approved July 27, 1861, the bounty due and remaining unpaid shall be credited upon their final statements, and be paid, like other arrearages, by the Pay Department.

II. The exercise of the powers given the Medical Inspectors of the army to discharge soldiers for disability, is suspended until their duties in this respect are defined by Regulations to be published hereafter.

III. Paragraph II. General Orders, No. 87 of 1863, is hereby modified so as to allow the Assistant Surgeon-General, Medical Inspector-General, and Medical Inspectors, the same number of rooms as offices, and fuel and furniture therefor, as are allowed by Regulations to officers of the Quartermaster's Department who have the same rank.

GENERAL ORDERS NO. 173.

War Department, Adjutant-General's Office,
Washington, *June* 11, 1863.

Hereafter in giving discharges to officers and soldiers, on account of disability, their discharge papers must always state whether, at the time of discharge, the officer or soldier was or was not physically suitable to enter or re-enlist in the Invalid Corps.

So much of General Orders No. 105, from this department, as forbids the "discharge of any man upon surgeon's certificate of disability who may be fit for service in the Invalid Corps" is so far modified as not to include officers.

GENERAL ORDERS NO. 179.

War Department, Adjutant-General's Office.
Washington, *June* 17, 1863.

II. From and after the 30th instant, the envelopes of all *official* communications addressed to the heads of bureaux of the War Department having the franking privilege, must be marked "official," with the signature thereto of the officer writing the communication. Postage stamps are not required on such communications.

GENERAL ORDERS NO. 206.

War Department, Adjutant-General's Office,
Washington, *July* 3, 1863.

The attention of Commanding Officers of regiments, battalions not included in regiments, independent companies or batteries. and detachments, surgeons in charge of hospitals or detachments, and all persons in the military service commanding or controlling commissioned officers or enlisted men on special or detached service, is directed to General Orders, No. 72, from this office, of March 24, 1863.

The "Reports of Deserters," therein called for, must be promptly and regularly forwarded as directed. *"Monthly Reports" will embrace only such desertions as may have occurred during the month, and will not be a consolidation of previous reports.*

GENERAL ORDERS NO. 212.

War Department, Adjutant-General's Office,
Washington, *July* 9, 1863.

I. The Invalid Corps will be organized in Companies of two classes or Battalions.

II. Those men enlisted in, or transferred to the Invalid Corps, who are most efficient and able-bodied, capable of using a musket, performing guard duty, making light marches, etc., etc., will be assigned to Companies of the First Battalion. Those of a minor degree of physical efficiency, or who possess special qualifications as cooks, nurses, or clerks, and whose services are required in hospitals, will be assigned to Companies of the Second Battalion.

III. Companies of the First Battalion will be employed mainly as provost-guards, and guards in cities, etc. They will be armed with muskets, and will not be liable to active campaigns with the field armies.

IV. Companies of the Second Battalion will be armed with side arms only, and will be employed in hospitals as cooks, nurses, clerks, orderlies, etc., and as guards to hospitals or other public buildings.

V. The rolls of men for the Invalid Corps, required by General Orders Nos. 105 and 173, current series, from this Department, will state in each case the nature of the disability and the Battalion for which the man is qualified.

VI. In all general hospitals and convalescent camps these rolls will be prepared and sent direct to the Provost-Marshal-General, immediately after each regular muster. Convalescents will be required to perform such hospital or military duty as they are capable of, until such time as the medical officer in charge can decide, finally, whether they are fit for duty with their regiments, for transfer to the First or Second Battalion of the Invalid Corps, or proper subjects for discharge on Surgeon's certificate.

VII. The physical examination of men for the Invalid Corps must be made by the Surgeon in charge before they are reported to the Provost-Marshal-General.

VIII. Officers of the Invalid Corps on duty in hospitals will be subordinate to the Surgeon in charge, and shall aid him in the performance of his administrative and executive duties, under the following and such other regulations as may hereafter be established:

1. The senior officer of the Invalid Corps on duty in a hospital shall have, under the direction of the Surgeon in charge, the immediate supervision of all matters connected with the police and discipline of the hospital.

2. He will have the clothing, arms, equipments, and descriptive rolls of patients carefully preserved, and will note on the descriptive rolls all payments made, or clothing issued while in hospital.

3. When a soldier is received into the hospital without his descriptive list, he will immediately report the fact to the soldier's Company Commander, who is hereby required to furnish, without delay, the descriptive roll and accounts of pay and clothing.

4. He will supervise the preparation of muster and pay rolls, descriptive rolls, and clothing accounts; of final statements of pay and clothing, and of the inventories and reports required by General Regulations concerning soldiers who die absent from their Companies.

5. He will keep a record of deaths and interments, and will see that the dead are properly buried, and that each grave is designated by a registered head-board. In the absence of a Chaplain, he will keep the Chaplain's register.

6. He will conduct all correspondence in relation to the descrip-

tive rolls, clothing, arms, equipments, and personal effects of soldiers.

7. He should reside within the hospital precincts, and shall visit every part of it daily.

IX. In executing the provisions of General Orders, No. 105, from this Department, in regard to the selection of men for the Invalid Corps, Medical Inspectors, Surgeons in charge of Hospitals, Camps, Regiments, or of Boards of Enrolment, Military Commanders, and all others required to make the physical examination of men for the Invalid Corps, will be governed in their decisions by the following lists of qualifications and disqualifications for admission into this Corps:

PHYSICAL INFIRMITIES THAT INCAPACITATE ENLISTED MEN FOR FIELD SERVICE, BUT DO NOT DISQUALIFY THEM FOR SERVICE IN THE INVALID CORPS.

1. Epilepsy, if the seizures do not occur more frequently than once a month, and have not impaired the mental faculties.

2. Paralysis, if confined to one upper extremity.

3. Hypertrophy of the heart, unaccompanied with valvular lesion. Confirmed nervous debility or excitability of the heart, with palpitation, great frequency of the pulse, and loss of strength.

4. Impeded respiration following injuries of the chest, pneumonia, or pleurisy. Incipient consumption.

5. Chronic dyspepsia or chronic diarrhœa, which has long resisted treatment. Simple enlargement of the liver or spleen, with tender or tumid abdomen.

6. Chronic disorders of the kidneys or bladder, without manifest organic disease, and which have not yielded to treatment. Incontinence of urine; mere frequency of micturition does not exempt.

7. Decided feebleness of constitution, whether natural or acquired. Soldiers over fifty and under eighteen years of age, are proper subjects for the Invalid Corps.

8. Chronic rheumatism, if manifested by positive change of structure, wasting or contraction of the muscles of the affected limb, or puffiness or distortion of the joints.

9. Pain, if accompanied with manifest derangement of the general health, wasting of a limb, or other positive sign of disease.

10. Loss of sight of right eye; partial loss of sight of both eyes, or permanent diseases of either eye, affecting the integrity or use of the other eye, vision being impaired to such a degree as clearly to incapacitate for field service. Loss of sight of left eye, or incurable diseases or imperfections of that eye, not affecting the use of the right eye, nor requiring medical treatment, do not disqualify for field service.

11. Myopia, if very decided or depending upon structural change of the eye. Hemeralopia, if confirmed.

12. Purulent otorrhœa; partial deafness, if in degree sufficient to prevent hearing words of command as usually given.

13. Stammering, unless excessive and confirmed.

14. Chronic aphonia, which has long resisted treatment, the voice remaining too feeble to give an order or an alarm, but yet sufficiently distinct for intelligible conversation.

15. Incurable deformities of either jaw, sufficient to impede but not to prevent mastication or deglutition. Loss of a sufficient number of teeth to prevent proper mastication of food.

16. Torticollis, if of long standing and well marked.

17. Hernia; abdomen grossly protuberant; excessive obesity.

18. Internal hæmorrhoids. Fistula in ano, if extensive or complicated, with visceral disease. Prolapsus ani.

19. Stricture of the urethra.

20. Loss or complete atrophy of both testicles from any cause; permanent retraction of one or both testicles within the inguinal canal.

21. Varicocele and circocele, if excessive or painful; simple sarcocele, if not excessive nor painful.

22. Loss of an arm, forearm, hand, thigh, leg, or foot.

23. Wounds or injuries of the head, neck, chest, abdomen, or back, that have impaired the health, strength, or efficiency of the soldier.

24. Wounds, fractures, injuries, tumors, atrophy of a limb, or chronic diseases of the joints or bones that would impede marching, or prevent continuous muscular exertion.

25. Anchylosis of the shoulder, elbow, wrist, knee, or ankle-joint.

26. Irreducible dislocation of the shoulder, elbow, wrist, or ankle-joint, in which the bones have accommodated themselves to their new relations.

27. Muscular or cutaneous contractions from wounds or burns, in a degree sufficient to prevent useful motion of a limb.

28. Total loss of a thumb, loss of ungual phalanx of right thumb; permanent contraction or extension of either thumb.

29. Total loss of any two fingers of the same hand.

30. Total loss of index finger of right hand; loss of second and third phalanges of index finger of right hand, if the stump is tender or the motion of the first phalanx is impaired. Loss of the third phalanx does not incapacitate for field service.

31. Loss of the second and third phalanges of all the fingers of either hand.

32. Permanent extension or permanent contraction of any finger, except the little finger; all the fingers adherent or united.

33. Total loss of either great toe; loss of any three toes on the same foot; all the toes joined together.

34. Deformities of the toes, if sufficient to prevent marching.

35. Large, flat, ill-shaped feet that do not come within the designation of talipes valgus, but are sufficiently malformed to prevent marching.

36. Varicose veins of inferior extremities, if large and numerous, having clusters of knots, and accompanied with chronic swellings.

37. Extensive, deep, and adherent cicatrices of lower extremities.

X. Soldiers having nervous debility or excitability of the heart, impeded respiration from curable causes, chronic dyspepsia, chronic diarrhœa, chronic disorders of the kidneys or bladder, incontinence of urine, aphonia, hemeralopia, or other disease or infirmity not incurable, are not to be recommended for the Invalid Corps until they have been under medical treatment or observation a sufficient length of time to make it extremely probable, if not certain, that they will not be fit for active field service during any considerable portion of their period of enlistment.

XI. Soldiers who have lost an arm, forearm, hand, thigh, leg, or foot, may be discharged from the army on Surgeon's certificate, if they so elect.

XII. None of the foregoing disabilities disqualify officers for service in the Invalid Corps, but some of them may be so aggravated or complicated as to unfit for any service. All such cases should be discharged.

XIII. In all cases where the physical infirmities of officers or enlisted men come within the provisions of the above list, they will be recommended for transfer to, or enlistment in, the Invalid Corps; but no one will be admitted into this Corps whose previous record does not show that he is meritorious and deserving, and that he has complied with the provisions of General Orders, No. 105, War Department, Adjutant-General's Office, 1863, authorizing an Invalid Corps.

PHYSICAL INFIRMITIES THAT DISQUALIFY ENLISTED MEN FOR SERVICE IN THE INVALID CORPS.

1. Manifest imbecility or insanity.

2. Epilepsy, if the seizures occur more frequently than once a month, and have obviously impaired the mental faculties.

3. Paralysis or chorea.

4. Organic diseases of the brain or spinal cord; of the heart or lungs; of the stomach or intestines; of the liver or spleen; of the kidneys or bladder, so extensive and long continued as to have seriously impaired the general health, or so well marked as to leave no reasonable doubt of the man's incapacity for service in the Invalid Corps.

5. Confirmed consumption, cancer, aneurism of important arteries.

6. Inveterate and extensive disease of the skin.

7. Scrofula, or constitutional syphilis, which has resisted treatment and seriously impaired the general health.

8. Habitual or confirmed intemperance, or solitary vice, sufficient in degree to have materially enfeebled the constitution.

9. Great injuries or diseases of the skull, occasioning impairment of the intellectual faculties, epilepsy, or other serious nervous or spasmodic symptoms.

10. Total loss of sight, partial loss of sight of both eyes, and permanent diseases of either eye affecting the integrity and use of the other eye, vision being so greatly impaired as to leave no reasonable doubt of the man's incapacity for service in the Invalid Corps.

11. Loss of nose, or deformity of nose, if sufficient seriously to obstruct respiration; ozœna, if dependent upon caries.

12. Deafness.

13. Dumbness, permanent loss of voice.

14. Total loss of tongue, partial loss, and hypertrophy or atrophy of tongue, if sufficient to make the speech unintelligible and prevent mastication or deglutition.

15. Incurable deformities of either jaw, whether congenital or produced by accident, which would prevent mastication or greatly injure the speech.

16. Tumors of the neck, impeding respiration or deglutition; fistula of larynx or trachea.

17. Deformity of the chest, sufficient to impede respiration or to prevent the carrying of arms and military equipments; caries of the ribs.

18. Artificial anus; severe stricture of the rectum.

19. Total loss, or nearly total loss, of penis; epispadia or hypospadia at the middle or nearer the root of the penis; stone in the bladder.

20. Incurable permanent organic stricture of the urethra, in which the urine is passed drop by drop, or which is complicated by disease of the bladder; urinary fistula.

21. Confirmed or malignant sarcocele; hydrocele, if complicated with organic disease of the testis.

22. Excessive anterior or posterior curvature of the spine; caries of the spine; lumbar abscess.

23. Anchylosis of the hip-joint.

24. Irreducible dislocation of hip or knee-joint.

25. Large chronic ulcers of lower extremities.

XIV. In all cases where the physical infirmities of an officer or enlisted man come within the provisions of this list, or where his previous record shows that he is not entitled to be received into the Invalid Corps, he will, if in service, be discharged; and if an applicant to reënter, his application will be disapproved.

XV. All orders or parts of orders inconsistent with the foregoing are revoked.

GENERAL ORDERS NO. 247.

War Department, Adjutant-General's Office,
Washington, *July* 29, 1863.

Section 8 of the Act of March 3, 1863, entitled "An Act to promote the Efficiency of the Corps of Engineers, etc.," reads thus:

SEC. 8. *And be it further enacted*, That the Officers of the Medical Department shall unite with the line officers of the army, under such rules and regulations as shall be prescribed by the Secretary of War, in supervising the cooking within the same, as an important sanitary measure; and that said Medical Department shall promulgate to its officers such regulations and instructions as may tend to insure the proper preparation of the ration of the soldier.

To meet the requirements of this enactment, the words "attended by the Senior Medical Officer of his command," in paragraph 116, Regulations 1861, will be inserted after the word "regiment," in the last sentence but one, so as to make that sentence read thus: "The Commanding Officer of the Post or Regiment, attended by the Senior Medical Officer of his command, will make frequent inspections of the kitchens or messes;" and the following will be added thereto: "The Medical Officer will submit his suggestions for improving the cooking, in writing, to the Commanding Officer."

GENERAL ORDERS No. 301.

War Department, Adjutant-General's Office,
Washington, *September* 7, 1863.

Under the provisions of section 42, Act of March 3, 1863, the head of each Bureau in each Executive Department is to be considered a part of the Executive Department, and letters written by an officer of the Government *on official business* to the Department, or to any head of a Bureau or Department, are to be passed free of postage. Such letters must be marked *official* on the envelope, with the official signature of the writer underneath.

GENERAL ORDERS NO. 308.

War Department, Adjutant-General's Office,
Washington, *September* 12, 1863.

The Medical Inspector-General has, under the direction of the Surgeon-General, the supervision of all that relates to the sanitary condition of the Army, whether in transports, quarters, or camps; the hygiene, police, discipline, and efficiency of field and general hospitals; and the assignment of duties to Medical Inspectors.

Medical Inspectors are charged with the duty of inspecting the sanitary condition of transports, quarters, and camps of field and general hospitals, and will report to the Medical Inspector-General all circumstances relating to the sanitary condition and wants of troops and of hospitals, and to the skill, efficiency, and conduct of the officers and attendants connected with the Medical Department. They are required to see that all regulations for protecting the health of troops, and for the careful treatment of and attendance upon the sick and wounded, are duly observed.

They will carefully examine into the quantity, quality, and condition of medical and hospital supplies, the correctness of all medical, sanitary, statistical, military, and property records and accounts pertaining to the Medical Department, and the punctuality with which reports and returns, required by Regulations, have been forwarded to the Surgeon-General.

They will ascertain the amount of disease and mortality among the troops, inquire into the causes, and the steps that may have been taken for its prevention or mitigation, indicating, verbally or in writing, to the medical officers such additional measures or precautions as may be requisite. When sanitary reforms, requiring the sanction and coöperation of military authority, are urgently demanded, they will report at once, in writing, to the officer commanding Corps, Department, or Division, the circumstances and necessities of the case, and the measures considered advisable for their relief, forwarding a duplicate of such reports to the Medical Inspector-General.

They will instruct and direct the medical officers in charge as to the proper measures to be adopted for the correction of errors and abuses, and, in all cases of conflict of views, authority, or instructions, with those of Medical Directors, will report the circumstances fully and promptly to the Medical Inspector-General for the Surgeon-General's orders.

Upon or near the beginning of each month, Medical Inspectors will make minute and thorough inspections of hospitals, barracks, camps, transports, &c., &c., within the districts to which they are assigned, in conformity with these instructions, and the forms for inspection reports furnished them.

Monthly inspection reports, in addition to remarks under the several heads, will also convey the fullest information in regard to the medical and surgical treatment adopted; the advantages or disadvantages of location, construction, general arrangement and administration of hospitals, camps, barracks; the necessity for improvement, alteration, or repair, with such recommendations as will most certainly conduce to the health and comfort of the troops, and the proper care and treatment of the sick and wounded. When alterations, improvements, or repairs, requiring the action of Heads of Bureaux, are considered essential, special reports, accompanied by plans and approximate estimates of quantities or cost, will be made.

Medical Inspectors will make themselves fully conversant with the regulations of the Subsistence Department in all that relates to issues to hospitals, whether general, field, division, or regimental, and will satisfy themselves by rigid examination of accounts and expenditures, that the fund accruing from retained rations is judiciously applied, and not diverted from its proper purposes through the ignorance or inattention of medical officers, giving such information and instruction on this subject as may be required. They will also give close attention to the supervision of cooking by the medical officer, whose duty it is, under the Act of Congress of March 3, 1863, and General Orders, No. 247, of 1863, to "submit his suggestions for improving the cooking, in writing, to the commanding officer," and to accompany him in frequent inspections of the kitchens and messes.

They will exercise sound discrimination in reporting "an officer of the Medical Corps as disqualified, by age or otherwise, for promotion to a higher grade, or unfitted for the performance of his professional duties," and be prepared to submit evidence of its correctness to the Medical Board, by whom the charge will be investigated.

Medical Inspectors are also charged with the duty of designating, to the surgeon in charge of general hospitals and convalescent camps, all soldiers who are in their opinion fit subjects for discharge on surgeon's certificate of disability, or sufficiently recovered to be able for duty. In all such cases they will direct the surgeon to discharge from service, in accordance with existing orders and regulations, or return to duty those so designated.

Official communications to the Medical Inspector-General will be directed to the Surgeon-General, U. S. A., and plainly addressed on the left-hand lower corner of envelope "For the Medical Inspector-General," the name and title of the writer being *written* under the words "Official Business."

It is expected that all commanding officers will afford every facility to Medical Inspectors in the execution of their important duties, giving such orders as may be necessary to carry into effect their suggestions and recommendations; and it is enjoined upon all medical officers, and others connected with the Medical Department of the United States Army, to yield prompt compliance with the instructions they may receive from Medical Inspectors on duty in the Army, Department, or District in which they are serving, on all matters relating to the sanitary condition of the troops, and of the hygiene, police, discipline, and efficiency of hospitals.

GENERAL ORDERS No. 316.

War Department, Adjutant-General's Office,
Washington, *September* 18, 1863.

Promotions and Appointments in the Army of the United States, made by the President, by and with the Advice and Consent of the Senate, and by the President alone, since the publication of General Orders No. 181, *of November* 1, 1862, *and up to July* 1, 1863. *Those made by the President alone are designated by a star.*

I. PROMOTIONS.—MEDICAL DEPARTMENT.

* Assistant-Surgeon James T. Ghiselin, to be Surgeon, June 14, 1862, *vice* Wood, appointed Assistant-Surgeon-General.

Assistant-Surgeon John F. Randolph, to be Surgeon, August 27, 1862, *vice* De Camp, retired.

Assistant-Surgeon George Hammond, to be Surgeon, August 27, 1862, *vice* Edgar, retired.

Assistant-Surgeon Anthony Heger, to be Surgeon, September 17, 1862, *vice* White, killed in battle.

* Assistant-Surgeon Charles T. Alexander, to be Surgeon, February 9, 1863, *vice* Barnes, appointed Medical Inspector.

* Assistant-Surgeon Bennett A. Clements, to be Surgeon, February 27, 1863, *vice* Summers, appointed Medical Inspector.

II. APPOINTMENTS.—MEDICAL DEPARTMENT.

To be Medical Inspectors, with the rank of Lieutenant-Colonel.

Surgeon Joseph K. Barnes, United States Army, February 9, 1863, to fill an original vacancy.

Surgeon Frank H. Hamilton, United States Volunteers, February 9, 1863, to fill an original vacancy.

Surgeon Peter Pineo, United States Volunteers, February 9, 1863, to fill an original vacancy.

Surgeon Augustus C. Hamlin, United States Volunteers, February 9, 1863, to fill an original vacancy.

George K. Johnson, of Michigan, February 9, 1863, to fill an original vacancy.

Surgeon John E. Summers, United States Army, February 27, 1863, to fill an original vacancy.

N. S. Townshend, of Ohio, March 11, 1863, to fill an original vacancy.

Surgeon George W. Stipp, United States Volunteers, March 12, 1863, to fill an original vacancy.

Charles C. Lee, of Pennsylvania, to be Assistant-Surgeon, November 22, 1862, *vice* Randolph, promoted.

Samuel H. Orton, of New Jersey, to be Assistant-Surgeon, November 22, 1862, *vice* Taylor, promoted.

John W. Brewer, of Maryland, to be Assistant-Surgeon, November 22, 1862, *vice* Hammond, promoted.

John Homans, Jr., of Massachusetts, to be Assistant-Surgeon, November 22, 1862, *vice* Bailey, retired.

John Brooke, of Pennsylvania, to be Assistant-Surgeon, November, 22, 1862, *vice* Irwin, promoted.

William H. Gardner, of the District of Columbia, to be Assistant-Surgeon, November 22, 1862, *vice* Heger, promoted.

* James Phillips, of Maryland, to be Assistant-Surgeon, November, 22, 1862. (Appointment since expired by constitutional limitation.)

* Harvey E. Brown, of New York, to be Assistant-Surgeon, April 13, 1863, *vice* Baxter, dismissed.

* J. Theodore Calhoun, of New Jersey, to be Assistant-Surgeon, April 13, 1863, *vice* Eastman, resigned.

* Edward J. Darken, of Connecticut, to be Assistant-Surgeon, April 13, 1863, *vice* Alexander, promoted.

* William E. Whitehead, of New Jersey, to be Assistant-Surgeon, April 13, 1863, *vice* Clements, promoted.

* William F. Norris, of Pennsylvania, to be Assistant-Surgeon, June 13, 1863, *vice* Craig, resigned.

* Edward Cowles, of Vermont, to be Assistant-Surgeon, June 13, 1863, *vice* Kennedy, resigned.

* Michael Hillary, of New York, to be Assistant-Surgeon, June 13, 1863, *vice* Pooley, resigned.

* William M. Giles, of New York, to be Medical Storekeeper, June 20, 1863, *vice* Zoeller, resigned.

TO BE SURGEONS OF VOLUNTEERS.

John Neil, of Pennsylvania, September 11, 1862.
James C. Whitehill, of Illinois, November 7, 1862.
Alexander B. Mott, of ——, November 7, 1862.
William M. Breed, of Pennsylvania, November 7, 1862 (since resigned).
Pliny A. Jewett, of Connecticut, November 7, 1862.
John J. Reese, of Pennsylvania, November 7, 1862.
John O. Bronson, of New York, November 7, 1862.
Augustus C. Bournonville, of Pennsylvania, November 7, 1862 (since resigned).
William S. Forbes, of Pennsylvania, November 7, 1862.
Thomas P. Gibbons, of Pennsylvania, November 7, 1862.
David Stanton, of Pennsylvania, November 7, 1862.
Frederick S. Ainsworth, of Massachusetts, November 7, 1862.
Francis Salter, of Ohio, November 7, 1862.
Howard Culbertson, of Ohio, November 7, 1862.
Augustus M. Clark, of New York, December 4, 1862.
Joseph H. Wythes, of Pennsylvania, December 4, 1862.
William Moss, of Pennsylvania, December 4, 1862.
Sylvanus S. Mulford, of New York, December 4, 1862.
E. D. Kittoe, of Illinois, December 4, 1862.
John Wilson, of Pennsylvania, December 4, 1862.
James W. Fitzpatrick, of New York, January 7, 1863.
George B. Twitchell, of New Hampshire, January 7, 1863.
William Goodell, of Pennsylvania, February 9, 1863.
Daniel G. Brinton, of Pennsylvania, February 9, 1863.
John E. Herbst, of Maryland, February 9, 1863.
Joseph S. Hildreth, of Massachusetts, February 9, 1863.
W. G. Varnum, of Missouri, February 9, 1863.
John H. Phillips, of New Jersey, February 9, 1863.
James M. McNulty, of California, February 19, 1863.
R. M. S. Jackson, of Pennsylvania, February 19, 1863.
Socrates N. Sherman, of Vermont, February 19, 1863.
John M. Robinson, of Ohio, February 19, 1863.
Adolf Majer, of New York, February 19, 1863.
Samuel B. Davis, of Kansas, February 19, 1863.
Ernst W. Thurm, of the District of Columbia, February 19, 1863.
Jacob R. Ludlow, of Maryland, February 19, 1863.
John B. Brumley, of New Jersey, February 19, 1863.
Charles Mayo, of the District of Columbia, February 19, 1863.
Ferdinand Hayden, of Pennsylvania, February 19, 1863.
Sanford B. Hunt, of Maryland, February 19, 1863.
William H. Gobrecht, of Pennsylvania, February 19, 1863.
George R. Weeks, of Ohio, February 19, 1863.

* Benjamin B. Wilson, of Pennsylvania, March 26, 1863.
* Henry Janes, of Vermont, March 26, 1863.
* Bernard J. Vanderkieft, of Maryland, March 26, 1863.
* Edward B. Dalton, of New York, March 26, 1863.
* William S. Thompson, of Pennsylvania, March 26, 1863.
* John W. Foye, of Massachusetts, March 26, 1863.
* Samuel D. Turney, of Ohio, March 26, 1863.
* George L Sutton, of New York, April 13, 1863.
* Andrew F. Sheldon, of New York, April 13, 1863.
* Peter H. Cleary, of New York, April 13, 1863.
* Robert R. Taylor, of Iowa, April 13, 1863.
* Caleb W. Horner, of Pennsylvania, April 13, 1863.
* Edward J. Whitney, of New York, April 13, 1863.
* Seymour D. Carpenter, of Iowa, April 13, 1863.
* Richard J. Lewis, of Pennsylvania, April 13, 1863.
* Robert S. Kenderdine, of Pennsylvania, April 13, 1863.
* John E. McDonald, of New York, April 13, 1863.
* Cyrus N. Chamberlin, of Massachusetts, April 13, 1863.
* William A. Conover, of New Jersey, May 8, 1863.
* Frederick A. Keffer, of Pennsylvania, May 8, 1863.
* Lewis D. Harlow, of Pennsylvania, May 8, 1863.
* Elmore Y. Chase, of Ohio, May 27, 1863.
* Conrad C. Dumreicher. of Illinois, May 27, 1863.
* David B. Sturgeon, of Pennsylvania, May 27, 1863.
* Henry A. Schlæfflin, of the District of Columbia, May 27, 1863.
* James W. Pettinos, of Pennsylvania, May 27, 1863.
* John Bradley, of Pennsylvania, June 13, 1863.
* Alexander M. Speer, of Pennsylvania, June 13, 1863.
* Robert Reyburn, of Pennsylvania, June 13, 1863.
* S. E. Fuller, of Connecticut, June 13, 1863.
* George F. French, of New Hampshire, June 13, 1863.
* Patrick A. O'Connell, of Massachusetts, June 13, 1863.
* John W. Lawton, of Massachusetts, June 29, 1863.
* St. John W. Mintzer, of Pennsylvania, June 29, 1863.
* Joseph B. Morrison, of Pennsylvania, June 29, 1863.
* Abraham M. Wilder, of Massachusetts, June 29, 1863.
* Philip Harvey, of Iowa, June 29, 1863.
* James B. Bellangee, of New Jersey, June 29, 1863.
* John L. Teed, of Illinois, June 29, 1863.
* Louis W. Reed, of Pennsylvania, June 29, 1863.

TO BE ASSISTANT-SURGEONS.

Samuel B. Davis, of Kansas, October 4, 1862 (since appointed Surgeon).

E. D. Kittoe, of Illinois, November 7, 1862 (since appointed Surgeon).

Lewis D. Harlow, of Pennsylvania, November 7, 1862 (since appointed Surgeon).

Edwin Freeman, of Ohio, November 7, 1862.

Edward J. Whitney, of New York, November 7, 1862 (since appointed Surgeon).

Mitchel H. Picot, of Pennsylvania, November 7, 1862 (since resigned).

Caleb W. Horner, of Pennsylvania, November 7, 1862 (since appointed Surgeon).

Charles E. Swasey, of New Hampshire, November 7, 1862.

William Watson, of Iowa, November 7, 1862.

Robert R. Taylor, of Ohio, November 7, 1862 (since appointed Surgeon).

Richard J. Lewis, of Pennsylvania, January 7, 1863 (since appointed Surgeon).

Robert S. Kenderdine, of Pennsylvania, January 7, 1863 (since appointed Surgeon).

John W. Lawton, of Massachusetts, January 7, 1863 (since appointed Surgeon).

Lewis J. Rice, of Pennsylvania, January 7, 1863.

Jacob J. De Lamater, of Pennsylvania, January 7, 1863.

Horatio B. Buck, of Maine, January 7, 1863.

Edward F. Bates, of New York, January 7, 1863.

Dennis B. Hannan, of Massachusetts, January 7, 1863.

St. John W. Mintzer, of Pennsylvania, January 7, 1863 (since appointed Surgeon).

Jacob W. Merriam, of New York, January 7, 1863.

Harley P. Mathewson, of Vermont, January 7, 1863.

James H. Peabody, of Maryland, January 7, 1863.

David S. Gloninger, of Pennsylvania, January 7, 1863.

Samuel D. Turney, of Ohio, February 19, 1863 (since appointed Surgeon).

Henry N. Fisher, of New York, February 19, 1863.

Joseph B. Morrison, of Pennsylvania, February 19, 1863 (since appointed Surgeon).

M. K. Moxley, of Ohio, February 19, 1863.

William W. Wythes, of Delaware, February 19, 1863.

Charles F. Haynes, of Maine, February 19, 1863.

Abel C. Benedict, of Connecticut, February 19, 1863.

James M. Laing, of New York, February 19, 1863.

Francis Greene, of New York, February 19, 1863.

William Grinstead, of Missouri, February 27, 1863.

Adam C. Swartzwelder, of Ohio, February 27, 1863.

John Q. Adams, of New York, February 27, 1863.

O. K. Reynolds, of Missouri, March 11, 1863.

Bernard J. Vanderkieft of Maryland, March 11, 1863 (since appointed Surgeon).

Edward B. Dalton, of Massachusetts, March 11, 1863 (since appointed Surgeon).

Abraham M. Wilder, of Massachusetts, March 11, 1863 (since appointed Surgeon).

David G. Rush, of Pennsylvania, March, 11, 1863.
Samuel Hart, of the District of Columbia, March 11, 1863.
James M. Boisnot, of Pennsylvania. March 11, 1863.
Franklin Grube, of Pennsylvania, March 11, 1863.
John Trenor, of New York, March 11, 1863.
* James H. Currey, of Maryland, March 27, 1863.
* Henry T. Legler, of New York, March 27, 1863.
* John Bradley, of Pennsylvania, March 27, 1863 (since appointed Surgeon).
* John E. McDonald, of New York, March 27, 1863 (since appointed Surgeon).
* Cyrus N. Chamberlain, of Pennsylvania, March 27, 1863 (since appointed Surgeon).
* Frank Meacham, of Massachusetts, April 23, 1863.
* William Threlkeld, of Kentucky, April 23, 1863.
Philip Harvey, of Iowa, April 23, 1863 (since appointed Surgeon).
* Henry A. Schlaefflin, of New York, May 14, 1863 (since appointed Surgeon).
* James W. Pettinos, of Pennsylvania, May 14, 1863 (since appointed Surgeon).
* William Carroll, of Pennsylvania, May 14, 1863.
* James B. Bellangee, of New Jersey, May 14, 1863 (since appointed Surgeon).
* W. O. McDonald, of New York, May 14, 1863.
* William A. Banks, of Maine, May 14, 1863.
* Charles A. Kipp, of New Jersey, May 14, 1863.
* Robert Reyburn, of Pennsylvania, June 4, 1863 (since appointed Surgeon).
* Stephen E. Fuller, of Connecticut, June 4, 1863 (since appointed Surgeon).
* George F. French. of New Hampshire, June 4, 1863 (since appointed Surgeon).
* William C. Bennett, of Connecticut, June 4, 1863.
* Patrick A. O'Connell, of Massachusetts, June 4, 1863 (since appointed Surgeon).
* John L. Teed, of Illinois, June 12, 1863 (since appointed Surgeon).
* Louis W. Reed, of Pennsylvania, June 23, 1863 (since appointed Surgeon).

V.—CASUALTIES.—RESIGNED (60).

Assistant-Surgeon James H. Pooley, April 27, 1863.
Assistant-Surgeon Lewis M. Eastman, January 19, 1863.
Hospital Chaplain S. Y. McMasters, March 25, 1863.
Hospital Chaplain Lyman N. Freeman, February 16, 1863.
Hospital Chaplain Joseph Aschwander, May 12, 1863.

Appointment which has expired by Constitutional Limitation, not having been Confirmed by the Senate (12).

James Phillips, as Assistant-Surgeon, March 4, 1863.

DISMISSED.

Assistant-Surgeon Andrew J. Baxter, January 19, 1863.

VI.—*Casualties in the Volunteer Force raised under the Acts approved July* 22 *and* 25, 1861, *and July* 5, 1838.

RESIGNED (130).

Surgeon Rufus K. Brown, December 10, 1862.
Surgeon Timothy Haynes, November 6, 1862.
Surgeon James King, November 6, 1862.
Surgeon William W. Strew, November 6, 1862.
Surgeon Samuel L. Bigelow, November 6, 1862.
Surgeon S. R. Haven, March 9, 1863.
Surgeon Rufus H. Johnson, January 8, 1863.
Surgeon James D. Robison, February 13, 1863.
Surgeon William W. Nassau, January 23, 1863.
Surgeon C. B. Chapman, March 24, 1863.
Surgeon Gaylord D. Beebe, March 9, 1863.
Surgeon Augustus C. Bournonville, March 23, 1863.
Surgeon William M. Breed, April 7, 1863.
Surgeon D. Hayes Agnew, April 7, 1863.
Surgeon Thomas G. Catlin, April 7, 1863.
Surgeon J. B. Peale, April 29, 1863.
Assistant-Surgeon Mitchel H. Picot, April 17, 1863.
Assistant-Surgeon John W. Brewer, November 26, 1862.

COMMISSIONS VACATED BY NEW APPOINTMENT.

By Medical Inspector Frank H. Hamilton, United States Army, his commission as Surgeon, United States Volunteers, February 9, 1863.

By Medical Inspector Peter Pineo, United States Army, his commission as Surgeon, United States Volunteers, February 9, 1863.

By Medical Inspector Augustus C. Hamlin, United States Army, his commission as Surgeon, United States Volunteers, February 9, 1863.

By Medical Inspector George W. Stipp, United States Army, his commission as Surgeon, United States Volunteers, March 12, 1863.

DECLINED (59).

By Alpheus B. Crosby, of New Hampshire, the appointment of Surgeon, April 4, 1862.

By William Goodell, of Pennsylvania, the appointment of Surgeon, February 9, 1863.

By John O. Bronson, of New York, the appointment of Assistant-Surgeon, September 11, 1862.

By Josiah Andrews, of ———, the appointment of Assistant-Surgeon, September 11, 1862.

By Samuel B. Davis, of ———, the appointment of Assistant-Surgeon, October 4, 1862.

By Adrian Woodward, of ———, the appointment of Assistant-Surgeon, November 7, 1862.

By Louis W. Read, of ———, the appointment of Assistant-Surgeon, November 7, 1862.

By William S. Edgar, of ———, the appointment of Assistant-Surgeon, November 7, 1862.

By H. M. Crawford, of ———, the appointment of Assistant-Surgeon, November 7, 1862.

By Roger W. Pease, of Maryland, the appointment of Assistant-Surgeon, February 19, 1863.

By James M. Boisnot, of Pennsylvania, the appointment of Assistant-Surgeon, March 11, 1863.

By H. W. Kendall, of ———, the appointment of Assistant-Surgeon, April 23, 1863.

By W. M. Smith, of ———, the appointment of Assistant-Surgeon, April 23, 1863.

By William Frothingham, of ———, the appointment of Assistant-Surgeon, January 7, 1863.

DIED (29).

Surgeon Samuel W. Everett, *killed at the battle of Shiloh, Tennessee*, April 6, 1862.

DROPPED (1).

Assistant-Surgeon George E. Pattee, October 14, 1862.

DISMISSED (7).

Surgeon Ferris Jacobs, December 22, 1862.
Surgeon George Burr, November 18, 1862.

DISCHARGED (17).

Surgeon George S. Kemble, February 10, 1863.
Surgeon Thomas McMartin, February 10, 1863.
Surgeon J. Taylor Bradford, February 19, 1863.
Surgeon A. B. Shipman, February 23, 1863.

GENERAL ORDERS NO. 326.

War Department, Adjutant-General's Office,
Washington, *Sept.* 28, 1863.

The attention of General Courts-Martial is directed to section 22 of the "Act for Enrolling and Calling out the National Forces, and for other Purposes," approved March 3, 1863, as follows:

"*And be it further enacted*, That courts-martial shall have power to sentence officers who shall absent themselves from their commands without leave, to be reduced to the ranks to serve three years or during the war."

GENERAL ORDERS NO. 351.

War Department, Adjutant-General's Office,
Washington, *October* 29, 1863.

The employment of women nurses in the U. S. General Hospitals will in future be strictly governed by the following rules:

1. Persons approved by Miss Dix, or her authorized agents, will receive from her, or them, "certificates of approval," which must be countersigned by Medical Directors upon their assignment to duty as nurses within their Departments.
2. Assignments of "women nurses" to duty in General Hospitals will only be made upon application by the Surgeons in charge, through Medical Directors, to Miss Dix or her agents, for the number they require, not exceeding one to every thirty beds.
3. No females, except Hospital Matrons, will be employed in General Hospitals, or, after December 31, 1863, borne upon the Muster and Pay Rolls, without such certificate of approval and regular assignment, unless specially appointed by the Surgeon-General.
4. Women nurses, while on duty in General Hospitals, are under the exclusive control of the senior medical officer, who will direct their several duties, and may be discharged by him when considered supernumerary, or for incompetency, insubordination, or violation of his orders. Such discharge, with the reasons therefor, being endorsed upon the certificate, will be at once returned to Miss Dix.

GENERAL ORDERS NO. 355.

War Department, Adjutant-General's Office,
Washington, *November* 4, 1863.

Medical Directors of armies in the field will forward, direct to the Surgeon-General at Washington, duplicates of their reports to their several Commanding Generals of the killed and wounded, after every engagement.

GENERAL ORDERS NO. 361.

War Department, Adjutant-General's Office,
Washington, *November* 9, 1863.

By direction of the President of the United States, Assistant-Surgeon *Benjamin King*, U. S. Army, is hereby retired from active service, and his name will be entered on the retired list of officers of the grade to which he now belongs, in accordance with section 12, Act approved July 17, 1862, he having been borne on the Army Register more than forty-five years.

GENERAL ORDERS NO. 390.

War Department, Adjutant-General's Office,
Washington, *December* 8, 1863.

Officers of the Medical Department, in charge of Hospitals for Blacks, are authorized to employ as cooks or nurses either males or females, who will be paid by the Medical Purveyor or Storekeeper at the rate of ten dollars per month.

In cases where white females are employed they will receive forty cents per day. All such persons will also receive one ration per day.

MEMORANDUM TO CORRECT GENERAL ORDERS, NO. 390, DATED WAR DEPARTMENT, ADJUTANT-GENERAL'S OFFICE, WASHINGTON, DECEMBER 8, 1863.

The employment of either males or females as cooks or nurses is authorized in *all* General Hospitals.

GENERAL ORDERS NO. 391.

War Department, Adjutant-General's Office,
Washington, *December* 9, 1863.

Commanders of Departments are authorized to grant furloughs to enlisted men in the General Hospitals within the limits of their command, upon the approval of the Medical Director or Chief Medical Officer. The number allowed to be absent at one time to be limited to five (5) per cent., and the period not to exceed thirty (30) days, and to be graduated according to the distance of the applicant from his home. The good conduct of the applicant to be made the rule of the Medical Officers in recommending the furloughs.

GENERAL ORDERS NO. 2.

War Department, Adjutant-General's Office,
Washington, *January* 2, 1864.

The percentage of men allowed to be absent at one time under the authority given in General Orders, No. 391, of 1863, to grant furloughs to enlisted men in hospitals, is changed from five to twenty per cent.

GENERAL ORDERS NO. 9.

War Department, Adjutant-General's Office,
Washington, *January* 4, 1864.

The Hospital and Ambulance Flags of the Army are established as follows: For General Hospitals, yellow bunting 9 by 5 feet, with the letter H, 24 inches long, of green bunting, in centre.

For Post and Field Hospitals, yellow bunting 6 by 4 feet, with letter H, 24 inches long, of green bunting, in centre.

For ambulances and guidons to mark the way to Field Hospitals, yellow bunting 14 by 28 inches, with a border, one inch deep, of green.

GENERAL ORDERS NO. 23.

War Department, Adjutant-General's Office,
Washington, *January* 16, 1864.

General Orders, No. 390, dated War Department, Adjutant-

General's Office, Washington, December 8, 1863, is hereby revoked, and the following substituted therefor:

The employment of persons of African descent, male or female, as cooks or nurses, will be permitted in all U. S. General Hospitals.

When so employed they will receive ten dollars per month and one ration. They will be paid by the nearest Medical Disbursing Officer, on rolls similar to those used in the payment of men of the Hospital Corps.

CIRCULAR.

War Department, Adjutant-General's Office,
Washington, *January* 18, 1864.

All invalid soldiers mustered on invalid transfer rolls by surgeons in charge of general hospitals, and all men of the 2d battalion companies who can be spared from the hospital, and who have so far recovered from their wounds or disease as to be thought fit for duty in the 1st battalion, will be sent to the invalid camp or depôt nearest to the hospital; and they will be there examined by a board, consisting of a field officer of the Invalid Corps and a medical officer of the regular or volunteer service, who shall have power to confirm their transfer to the corps, and to decide to which battalion they shall be assigned; to send those judged fit for field duty to their regiments, and to discharge those whose infirmities unfit them for any duty.

CIRCULAR NO. 11.

War Department, Adjutant-General's Office,
Washington, *January* 26, 1864.

The following instructions from the Secretary of War are furnished for your information and guidance:

The authority heretofore given to Military Commanders to order the discharge of enlisted men for disability is hereby revoked, and hereafter all discharges of Regulars (except rejected recruits, whose cases are forwarded to this office), and all discharges of Volunteers, except recruits rejected at the muster-in (who are discharged by the Mustering Officer, and called "rejected recruits"), will be given ONLY on the order of the Commanding Officer of the Corps or Department in which the man may be serving at the time of discharge. This will not be understood to confer upon Corps or Department Commanders authority to grant discharges to enlisted men, except by Orders from the War Department, to accept promotion, or expiration of term of service, for disability, or by sentence of a General Court-Martial. Officers and soldiers of the Volunteer Force, discharged on expiration of term of service, should be mustered out of service by the Commissary or Assistant-Commissary of Musters for their command.

GENERAL ORDERS NO. 47.

War Department, Adjutant-General's Office,
Washington, *February* 5, 1864.

All medical and hospital supplies and property in possession of officers of the Quartermaster's Department on the Mississippi river and its tributaries, for storage or safe-keeping, that have been unclaimed for three months, will at once be forwarded to the nearest Medical Purveyors, with invoices setting forth the number of packages, from whom, and when received. Duplicates of the invoices will be sent to the Surgeon-General of the Army.

GENERAL ORDERS NO. 54.

War Department, Adjutant-General's Office,
Washington, *February* 12, 1864.

Medical Inspectors are authorized to inspect, condemn, and recommend for final disposition, such articles of Medical and Hospital property as may be regarded as useless and unfit for issue. They are the "Authorized Inspectors" for such property, under paragraphs 1022 and 1023, General Regulations for the Army.

GENERAL ORDERS NO. 55.

War Department, Adjutant-General's Office,
Washington, *February* 12, 1864.

Upon the death of a Commissioned Officer, in a general hospital, the Surgeon in charge, besides forwarding to the Adjutant-General the required inventory of his effects, will immediately inform the nearest relative of the officer what effects were left by him. If at the expiration of two months the articles are not called for by a person authorized to receive them, they will be sold at auction, and the proceeds sent to the Treasury, as prescribed by Regulations for the effects of enlisted men. Swords, watches, trinkets, and articles of that class will not be disposed of in this manner, but will be properly labelled with the name, rank, and regiment, and date of death of the owner, and sent to the Adjutant-General's Office, to be deposited with the Second Auditor of the Treasury to await the application of the heirs.

GENERAL ORDERS NO. 108.

War Department, Adjutant-General's Office,
Washington, *March* 15, 1864.

PAY OF OFFICERS RESIGNING OR DISMISSED.

1. An officer *on leave* who resigns, will be paid to the date given in the acceptance of his resignation.

2. An officer *on duty* who resigns, will be paid to the date at which he received notice of the acceptance of his resignation, provided he continued on duty till that time; otherwise, to the date when he was relieved from duty.

3. An officer *on leave* when he is dropped or dismissed from the military service, will be paid to the date inclusive of the order dropping or dismissing him, provided no other time be specified in the order as the date when his pay should cease, or when he ceased to be an officer, and, in such case, to the date so specified.

4. An officer *on duty* or in hospital when he is dropped or dismissed from the military service, will be paid to the date at which the order dropping or dismissing him was received at his post or

hospital, if no other time be specified in the order as the date when he ceased to be an officer, and, in such case, to the date so specified.

5. An officer dismissed by sentence of Court-Martial will be paid to the date when the order approving the sentence was received at the post where the officer was, if no other time be specified in the sentence, or in the order promulgating it, as the termination of his service and pay.

GENERAL ORDERS NO. 106.

War Department, Adjutant-General's Office,
Washington, *March* 16, 1864.

UNIFORM SYSTEM OF AMBULANCES.

The following Act of Congress is published for the information and guidance of all concerned:

PUBLIC.—NO. 22.

AN ACT to Establish a Uniform System of Ambulances in the Armies of the United States.

Be it enacted by the Senate and House of Representatives of the United States of America in Congress assembled, That the medical director, or chief medical officer, of each army corps shall, under the control of the medical director of the army to which such army corps belongs, have the direction and supervision of all ambulances, medicine, and other wagons, horses, mules, harness, and other fixtures appertaining thereto, and of all officers and men who may be detailed or employed to assist him in the management thereof, in the army corps in which he may be serving.

SEC. 2. *And be it further enacted*, That the commanding officer of each army corps shall detail officers and enlisted men for service in the ambulance corps of such army corps, upon the following basis, viz. one captain, who shall be commandant of said ambulance corps, one first lieutenant for each division in such army corps; one second lieutenant for each brigade in such army corps; one sergeant for each regiment in such army corps; three privates for each ambulance, and one private for each wagon; and the officers and non-commissioned officers of the ambulance corps shall be mounted: *Provided*, That the officers, non-commissioned officers, and privates so detailed for each army corps shall be examined by a board of medical officers of such army corps as to their fitness for such duty; and that such as are found to be not qualified shall be rejected, and others detailed in their stead.

SEC. 3. *And be it further enacted*, That there shall be allowed and furnished to each army corps two-horse ambulances, upon the following basis, to wit, three to each regiment of infantry of five hundred men or more; two to each regiment of infantry of more than two hundred and less than five hundred men or more; and one to each regiment of infantry of less than two hundred men; two to each regiment of cavalry of five hundred men or more;

and one to each regiment of cavalry of less than five hundred men; one to each battery of artillery—to which battery of artillery it shall be permanently attached; to the head-quarters of each army corps two such ambulances; and to each division train of ambulances two army wagons; and ambulances shall be allowed and furnished to division brigades and commands not attached to any army corps upon the same basis, and each ambulance shall be provided with such number of stretchers and other appliances as shall be prescribed by the Surgeon-General: *Provided*, That the ambulances and wagons herein mentioned shall be furnished, so far as practicable, from the ambulances and wagons now in the service.

SEC. 4. *And be it further enacted*, That the horse and mule litters may be adopted or authorized by the Secretary of War, in lieu of ambulances, when judged necessary, under such rules and regulations as may be prescribed by the medical director of each army corps.

SEC. 5. *And be it further enacted*, That the captain shall be the commander of all the ambulances, medicine, and other wagons in the corps, under the immediate direction of the medical director, or chief medical officer, of the army corps to which the ambulance corps belongs. He shall pay special attention to the condition of the ambulances, wagons, horses, mules, harness, and other fixtures appertaining thereto, and see that they are at all times in readiness for service; that the officers and men of the ambulance corps are properly instructed in their duties, and that their duties are performed, and that the regulations which may be prescribed by the Secretary of War, or the Surgeon-General, for the government of the ambulance corps are strictly observed by those under his command. It shall be his duty to institute a drill in his corps, instructing his men in the most easy and expeditious manner of moving the sick and wounded, and to require in all cases that the sick and wounded shall be treated with gentleness and care, and that the ambulances and wagons are at all times provided with attendants, drivers, horses, mules, and whatever may be necessary for their efficiency; and it shall be his duty also to see that the ambulances are not used for any other purpose than that for which they are designed and ordered. It shall be the duty of the medical director, or chief medical officer of the army corps, previous to a march, and previous to and in time of action, or whenever it may be necessary to use the ambulances, to issue the proper orders to the captain for the distribution and management of the same, for collecting the sick and wounded and conveying them to their destination. And it shall be the duty of the captain faithfully and diligently to execute such orders. And the officers of the ambulance corps, including the medical director, shall make such reports, from time to time, as may be required by the Secretary of War, the Surgeon-General, the medical director of the army, or the commanding officer of the army corps in which they may be serving; and all reports to higher authority than the commanding officer of the army corps shall be transmitted through the medical director of the army to which such army corps belongs.

Sec. 6. *And be it further enacted*, That the first lieutenant assigned to the ambulance corps for a division shall have complete control, under the captain of his corps and the medical director of the army corps, of all the ambulances, medicine, and other wagons, horses, mules, and men in that portion of the ambulance corps. He shall be the acting assistant-quartermaster for that portion of the ambulance corps, and will receipt for and be responsible for all the property belonging to it, and be held responsible for any deficiency in anything appertaining thereto. He shall have a travelling cavalry forge, a blacksmith, and a saddler, who shall be under his orders, to enable him to keep his train in order. He shall have authority to draw supplies from the depôt quartermaster, upon requisitions approved by the captain of his corps, the medical director, and the commander of the army corps to which he is attached. It shall be his duty to exercise a constant supervision over his train in every particular, and keep it at all times ready for service.

Sec. 7. *And be it further enacted*, That the second lieutenant shall have command of the portion of the ambulance corps for a brigade, and shall be under the immediate orders of the first lieutenant, and he shall exercise a careful supervision over the sergeants and privates assigned to the portion of the ambulance corps for his brigade; and it shall be the duty of the sergeants to conduct the drills and inspections of the ambulances, under his orders, of their respective regiments.

Sec. 8. *And be it further enacted*, That the ambulances in the armies of the United States shall be used only for the transportation of the sick and wounded, and, in urgent cases only, for medical supplies, and all persons shall be prohibited from using them, or requiring them to be used, for any other purpose. It shall be the duty of the officers of the ambulance corps to report to the commander of the army corps any violation of the provisions of this section, or any attempt to violate the same. And any officer who shall use an ambulance, or require it to be used, for any other purpose than as provided in this section, shall, for the first offence, be publicly reprimanded by the commander of the army corps in which he may be serving, and for the second offence shall be dismissed from the service.

Sec. 9. *And be it further enacted*, That no person except the proper medical officers, or the officers, non-commissioned officers, and privates of the ambulance corps, or such persons as may be specially assigned, by competent military authority, to duty with the ambulance corps for the occasion, shall be permitted to take or accompany sick or wounded men to the rear, either on the march or upon the field of battle.

SEC. 10. *And be it further enacted*, That the officers, non-commissioned officers, and privates of the ambulance corps shall be designated by such uniform or in such manner as the Secretary of War shall deem proper: *Provided*, That officers and men may be relieved from service in said corps and others detailed to the same, subject to the examination provided in the second section of this act, in the discretion of the commanders of the armies in which they may be serving.

SEC. 11. *And be it further enacted*, That it shall be the duty of the commander of the army corps to transmit to the Adjutant-General the names and rank of all officers and enlisted men detailed for service in the ambulance corps of such army corps, stating the organizations from which they may have been so detailed; and if such officers and men belong to volunteer organizations, the Adjutant-General shall thereupon notify the governors of the several States in which such organizations were raised, of their detail for such service; and it shall be the duty of the commander of the army corps to report to the Adjutant-General from time to time the conduct and behavior of the officers and enlisted men of the ambulance corps, and the Adjutant-General shall forward copies of such reports, so far as they relate to officers and enlisted men of volunteer organizations, to the governors of the States in which such organizations were raised.

SEC. 12. *And be it further enacted*, That nothing in this act shall be construed to diminish or impair the rightful authority of the commanders of armies, army corps, or separate detachments, over the medical and other officers and the non-commissioned officers and privates of their respective commands.

Approved March 11, 1864.

GENERAL ORDERS No. 107.

War Department, Adjutant-General's Office,
Washington, *March* 16, 1864.

CLOTHING OF SMALL-POX PATIENTS.

Hereafter, upon the discharge of soldiers from small-pox hospitals, the following articles of clothing will be issued to them gratuitously by the Quartermaster's Department:

1 pair trowsers, 1 blouse, 1 shirt, 1 pair drawers, 1 pair socks, 1 cap.

The infected clothing belonging to the men will be burned.

GENERAL ORDERS No. 127.

War Department, Adjutant-General's Office,
Washington, *March* 29, 1864.

I. Medical Directors of Departments will establish a General Hospital at some convenient point within their respective Departments, for the reception and treatment of sick and wounded officers, but no expenditures for the construction of new hospitals for this purpose will be incurred without special authority. They will detail a Surgeon-in-Charge, who will make requisitions upon the

Medical Purveyor for medicines, hospital stores, furniture, &c., according to the standard Supply Table of the Medical Department, and will hire the nurses, cooks, and laundresses required. Hospital Stewards assigned to Officers' General Hospitals will be paid on the regular muster and pay rolls.

II. On the recommendation of the Medical Director of the Department, a commissioned medical officer will be detailed to act permanently as Treasurer for each Officers' General Hospital, who shall not be removed without sufficient cause. The Treasurer shall have the custody of the funds of the Hospital, and shall perform such duties in relation to collecting, disbursing, and accounting for the same, and such other duties as may be prescribed by the Surgeon-General.

III. On the last day of each calendar month, and immediately on leaving the Hospital, by return to duty, furlough, or otherwise, each officer shall pay to the Treasurer the sum of one dollar for each and every day he has been in the Hospital, and for which he has not already paid as herein provided. When an officer has employed a special attendant, he shall pay thirty cents a day additional for each day such attendant was subsisted in the Hospital. Company officers of volunteers, while in such Officers' General Hospital, shall be considered as "on detached service without troops," for the purpose of drawing their pay and settling their indebtedness to the Hospital, and may be paid on separate pay accounts, instead of on the muster and pay rolls.

IV. When an officer is not provided with money, and is unable to obtain it, he will give a certificate of indebtedness, in triplicate, to the Treasurer of the Hospital, in such form as shall be prescribed by the Surgeon-General, for the amount due from him to the Hospital. The Treasurer shall immediately forward, for stoppage, two copies of the certificate to the Chief Paymaster of the Pay District in which the Hospital may be located, retaining the remaining copy for his own reference and security. When an officer is discharged from the Hospital to return to a regiment serving beyond the limits of the Pay District in which such Hospital is located, the Treasurer shall forward the certificates of indebtedness which the officer may have given to the proper Chief Paymaster, if known to him; otherwise, to the Paymaster-General, for such reference.

V. The Chief Paymaster of the Pay District will immediately cause the certificates of indebtedness to be placed in the hands of the Paymaster of the Hospital (or of the regiment, should the officer have left the Hospital), with instructions to stop the amounts on the first payment of the officers by whom the certificates were given. The Paymaster will take the receipt of each officer for the full amount of his pay account, and transmit the deducted sums to the Treasurer of the Hospital to which they are due, who will endorse receipt therefor upon the duplicate certificates in the Paymaster's hands, or furnish duplicate abstracts of receipts signed by him, and embracing in one receipt the names of all the officers on whose accounts the sums have been remitted. The Paymaster will also forward monthly an abstract of certificates thus paid to the Surgeon-General.

VI. Officers of the Subsistence Department will make *separate* abstracts of the sales to each Officers' General Hospital during each calendar month, and will report the same to the Commissary-General of Subsistence in the manner provided by regulations in relation to sales to officers. Payment for stores thus purchased of the Subsistence Department shall be made by the Treasurer monthly, and in cash, when practicable; but when the Treasurer has not money on hand sufficient to liquidate the entire indebtedness of the Hospital to the Subsistence Department, he shall give to the Commissary accountable for the stores sold a certificate of indebtedness, in duplicate, for the amount remaining unpaid, which certificate shall be a valid claim against the Hospital, and be paid from the first moneys received thereafter by the Treasurer, and until paid shall be considered as a sufficient cash voucher to the Commissary for the amount stated therein. When the Treasurer pays his certificate of indebtedness, he shall take the receipt of the Commissary for the amount thus paid him, and shall report his action in this matter to the Commissary-General of Subsistence, stating the date and amount of each certificate thus cancelled, the name of the Commissary receiving the money therefor, etc.

VII. Medical Directors of Armies in the field, when necessary, will establish temporary Hospitals in the rear of such armies, to be governed by the following regulations:

Medical Directors of Armies and of Departments and Medical Inspectors will frequently inspect Officers' General Hospitals, and in addition to the usual course of hospital inspection they will investigate the manner in which the Treasurer performs his duties, and promptly report any neglect on his part to the Surgeon-General.

VIII. No officer whose certificate of indebtedness to a Hospital remains unpaid by him shall receive pay without deducting therefrom the amount of this indebtedness and leaving it in the hands of the Paymaster, who shall give him duplicate receipts therefor, one of which the officer shall immediately forward to the Treasurer of the Hospital for which the stoppage is made. A violation of this paragraph will subject the officer so offending to court-martial for disobedience of orders.

IX. When an officer dies in Hospital, the Treasurer shall immediately ascertain the amount of his indebtedness to the Hospital, and prepare an account thereof in triplicate, which shall be certified to be correct by both the Treasurer and the Surgeon-in-Charge. One copy of this account shall be retained by the Treasurer, and the remaining two copies be forwarded to the Second Auditor of the Treasury, in order that, upon the final settlement of the officer's accounts, the amount of his indebtedness may be deducted from any pay due him, and remitted to the Treasurer of the Hospital.

GENERAL ORDERS No. 129.

War Department, Adjutant-General's Office,
Washington, *March* 30, 1864.

The attention of all officers is called to the Army Regulations and General Orders in regard to correspondence on official matters. All such correspondence must be conducted through the proper official channels, except in cases of pressing necessity, which do not leave time for regular communication, and then the necessity must be stated. All applications or correspondence, through whomsoever made, in violation of this order, will not be responded to, and the writers will be arrested and tried for disobedience of orders, or recommended to the President for dismissal.

GENERAL ORDERS No. 158.

War Department, Adjutant-General's Office,
Washington, *April* 13, 1864.

The following Act of Congress is published for the information of all concerned:

PUBLIC—NO. 44.

An Act to Amend Section Nine of the Act approved July Seventeenth, Eighteen Hundred and Sixty-two, entitled "An Act to define the Pay and Emoluments of certain Officers of the Army, and for other Purposes."

Be it enacted by the Senate and House of Representatives of the United States of America in Congress assembled, That the rank of Chaplain, without command, in the Regular and Volunteer service of the United States, is hereby recognised. Chaplains shall be borne on the field and staff rolls next after the Surgeons, and shall wear such uniform as is or may be prescribed by the Army Regulations, and shall be subject to the same rules and regulations as other officers of the army. They shall be entitled to draw forage for two horses, and when assigned to hospitals, posts, and forts, they shall be entitled to quarters and fuel within the hospitals, posts, or forts, while they are so assigned, without the privilege of commutation, subject to the same conditions and limitations as are now by law provided in the case of Surgeons. When absent from duty with leave, or on account of sickness or other disability, or when held by the enemy as prisoners, they shall be subject to no other diminution or loss of pay and allowances than other officers in the military service are under like circumstances. And Chaplains who have been absent from duty by reason of wounds or sickness, or when held as prisoners in the hands of the enemy, shall be entitled to receive full pay, without rations, during such absence. In all other respects the pay of Chaplains shall be the same as now provided by law.

SEC. 2. *And be it further enacted*, That the act approved July fourteenth, eighteen hundred and sixty two, entitled "An Act to grant Pensions," is hereby so amended as to include Chaplains in the Regular and Volunteer forces of the army: *Provided*, That the pension to which a Chaplain shall be entitled for a total disability shall be twenty dollars per month, and all the provisions of the act to which this section is an amendment shall apply to and embrace the widows, children, mothers, and sisters of Chaplains of the land forces who have died since the fourth day of March, eighteen hundred and sixty-one, or shall die, of wounds or disease contracted in the service of the United States, and while such Chaplains are, or shall be, in the line of their duty.

SEC. 3. *And be it further enacted*, That it shall be the duty of Chaplains in the military service of the United States to make monthly reports to the Adjutant-General of the army, through the usual military channels, of the moral condition and general history of the regiments, hospitals, or posts to which they may be attached; and it shall be the duty of all commanders of regiments, hospitals, and posts, to render such facilities as will aid in the discharge of the duties assigned to them by the Government.

SEC. 4. *And be it further enacted*, That all Chaplains in the military service of the United States shall hold appropriate religious services at the burial of soldiers who may die in the command to which they are assigned to duty, and it shall be their duty to hold public religious services at least once each Sabbath, when practicable.

Approved April 9, 1864.

GENERAL ORDERS NO. 177.

War Department, Adjutant-General's Office,
Washington, *April* 23, 1864.

IN RELATION TO PUBLIC HORSES, WAGONS, &C.

I. Every officer of the army, other than those of the Quartermaster's Department, and the chief medical officer of departments, armies, and army corps, who has in his possession, or under his control any horse, ambulance, spring wagon, or vehicle of any kind, belonging to the Government of the United States, whether used in the performance of his public or private duties, will immediately turn in the same to the Quartermaster's Department.

II. Hereafter no officer of the army will use any horse, ambulance, spring wagon, or vehicle of any kind, which is the property of the Government of the United States, whether for the transaction of his official or private business, without an order in writing from the Adjutant-General authorizing such use.

This order will not apply to officers entitled to be mounted under General Orders, No. 277, from this office, of August 8, 1863.

GENERAL ORDERS No. 198.

War Department, Adjutant-General's Office,
Washington, *May* 12, 1864.

DUTIES OF ASSISTANT SURGEON-GENERAL.

To facilitate the prompt transmission of medical supplies to points developed by emergencies, secure the proper distribution and presence of medical officers and their assistants where their services are most required, and to provide comfortable, abundant, and available hospital accommodation for the sick and wounded of the Armies of the West and Southwest, the office of the Assistant Surgeon-General is established at Louisville, Ky.

To fully accomplish these important objects, Assistant Surgeon-General R. C. Wood will have immediate control, under the general direction of the Surgeon-General, of the Medical affairs in the Military Department of the Northwest, the Northern Department, the Departments of Kansas, Missouri, and those composing the Division of the Mississippi, except that officers assigned to duty with any Army or Department will not be removed therefrom, unless by order of the War Department.

The orders, circulars, and instructions heretofore published by the Assistant Surgeon-General, and such as may in future be required, will be obeyed and respected by all under his jurisdiction.

GENERAL ORDERS No. 213.

War Department, Adjutant-General's Office,
Washington, *June* 18, 1864.

I. All sick and wounded officers absent from their commands and not fit for duty in the field, but able to sit on Courts-Martial, will immediately report their names and address to the Adjutant-General of the Army.

II. All staff and regimental medical officers now on leave in the Department of the East, in New Jersey, the eastern part of Pennsylvania, and the eastern part of Maryland, if able to travel, will report to the nearest Medical Director for examination; and those found unfit for active service, but able to do hospital duty, will be ordered to report immediately at the hospital at Camp Parole, near Annapolis, Maryland, for such duty as the Surgeon in charge may require of them.

GENERAL ORDERS NO. 216.

War Department, Adjutant-General's Office,
Washington, *June* 22, 1864.

The following Act of Congress is published for the information of all concerned:

PUBLIC—NO. 122.

AN ACT to increase the Pay of Soldiers in the United States Army, and for other Purposes.

SEC. 1. *Be it enacted by the Senate and House of Representatives of the United States of America in Congress assembled*, That on and after the first day of May, eighteen hundred and sixty-four, and during the continuance of the present rebellion, the pay per month of non-commissioned officers and privates in the military service of the United States shall be as follows, viz. hospital stewards of the first class, thirty-three dollars; hospital stewards of the second class, twenty-five dollars; hospital stewards of the third class, twenty-three dollars.

SEC. 11. *And be it further enacted*, That the thirty-first section of an act entitled "An Act for enrolling and calling out the National Forces, and for other Purposes," approved March third, one thousand eight hundred and sixty-three, be, and the same is hereby, so amended as that an officer may have, when allowed by order of his proper commander, leave of absence for other cause than sickness or wounds, without deduction from his pay or allowances. *Provided*, That the aggregate of such absence shall not exceed thirty days in any one year.

GENERAL ORDERS NO. 222.

War Department, Adjutant-General's Office,
Washington, *July* 4, 1864.

Medical Directors of armies *in the field* are authorized to employ, under contract as "Acting Staff Surgeons," Regimental Surgeons of two years' experience, who are specially recommended by their Medical Directors, and whose term of service has expired.

The rate of compensation will be the same as pay and emoluments of Regimental Surgeons, with use of one public horse and equipments and forage for the same.

PART IV.

CIRCULAR NO. 1.

Surgeon-General's Office,
Washington, D. C., *May* 5, 1862.

Medical officers will account semi-annually (June 30th and December 31st) to the Chief Medical Director of the Military Department in which they are serving, for all the medical and hospital property in their possession, and also to this office.

They will make at the same time, to the Surgeon-General, a "Semi-Annual Return of Knapsacks," stating their condition and from whom received.

WILLIAM A. HAMMOND,
Surgeon-General, U. S. Army.

CIRCULAR NO. 2.

Surgeon-General's Office,
Washington, D. C., *May* 21, 1862.

In the Monthly Reports of Sick and Wounded, the following details will be briefly mentioned in accompanying remarks:

SURGERY.

Fractures.—The date of reception, the situation, character, direction, treatment, and result in all cases.

Gunshot Wounds.—The date of reception, the situation, direction, and character, the foreign matters extracted (if any), and the result in all cases.

Amputations.—The period and nature of the injury, the character of the operation, the time, place, and result.

Exsections.—All operations for, with a statement of the injury demanding them, the date of injury, the date of operation, the joint or bone operated upon, and the result.

MEDICINE.

Fevers.—Their character and symptoms, an outline of the plans of treatment found most efficient, with remarks on the location and sanitary condition of camps, or quarters, during the prevalence of these disorders.

Diarrhœa and Dysentery.—Grade and treatment, with remarks on the character of the ration, and the modes of cooking.

Scorbutic Diseases.—Character and symptoms, with observations on causation, and a statement of the means employed to procure exemption.

Respiratory Diseases.—Symptoms, severity, and treatment, with remarks on the sheltering of the troops, and the atmospheric conditions.

Similar remarks on other preventible diseases.

Important cases of every kind should be reported in full. Where post-mortem examinations have been made, accounts of the pathological results should be carefully prepared.

As it is proposed to establish in Washington an *Army Medical Museum*, medical officers are directed diligently to collect and to forward to the office of the Surgeon-General, all specimens of morbid anatomy, surgical or medical, which may be regarded as valuable; together with projectiles and foreign bodies removed, and such other matters as may prove of interest in the study of military medicine or surgery.

These objects should be accompanied by short explanatory notes.

Each specimen in the collection will have appended the name of the medical officer by whom it was prepared.

WILLIAM A. HAMMOND,
Surgeon-General, U. S. Army.

NOTE.—Medical Directors will furnish one copy of this circular to every medical officer in the department in which they are serving; and they will hereafter forward to this office with their consolidated monthly reports, all the monthly reports of the medical officers under their supervision. They will also immediately transmit all back monthly reports, and papers of every kind relating to the above subjects of medicine and surgery, which may have accumulated in their respective offices since the commencement of the rebellion.

CIRCULAR NO. 4.

Surgeon-General's Office,
Washington, D.C., *June* 5, 1862.

The Secretary of War having authorized, in certain cases, the employment of civilians as cooks and nurses for duty in General Hospitals (only), the following rules and instructions are published for the information of all concerned:

REGULATONS FOR THE HOSPITAL CORPS OF THE UNITED STATES ARMY.

The men of the Hospital Corps will each receive $20.50 per month, besides clothing, rations, and medical attendance.

They will be under military discipline, and subject only to the orders of the medical authorities, and will wear the undress uniform of a private soldier, with a green half-chevron on the left forearm.

Their duties will be either nursing the sick and wounded of the army in hospitals, cooking, or any other duties with the sick at the discretion of the Medical Officers.

They will be divided into squads of eleven, one of whom will be responsible for the efficiency of the rest. One squad will be allowed to every one hundred patients.

At the usual roll-calls, the chief of the squad will answer for the rest to the Hospital Steward, who will thus learn the number of vacant beds in each ward, and all other particulars concerning the condition and wants of the hospital, which he will report to the Medical "Officer of the Day." The term of the service of the Hospital Corps will be according to the necessities of the service, or during good conduct.

The amount of pay and clothing received by each nurse, with date, will be recorded on their contract, which will be as a descriptive list to go with the nurse.

The senior Medical Officer in charge will make a monthly payroll of the Hospital Corps, similar to form 12, Medical Regulations, except the rank and designation, and transmit the same for payment to the nearest Medical Disbursing Officer.

Surgeons in charge of General Hospitals, when so authorized, may make con racts with persons for such service according to the provisions set forth herein.

WILLIAM A. HAMMOND,
Surgeon-General, U. S. Army.

NOTE.—It is hereby enjoined upon all Medical Officers that they shall not avail themselves of this special authority of the War Department without first receiving permission of the Surgeon-General to do so, on making a full statement of the facts in the case, and clearly setting forth the reasons why the permission should be granted, except in cases of immediate necessity and urgency, and then the Commanding Officer must approve. In such exceptional cases the facts will be promptly reported to the Surgeon-General with the necessary explanations, together with a request that permission be given to continue the employment if the necessity still exists.

CIRCULAR NO. 5.

Surgeon-General's Office,
Washington, D.C., *June* 9, 1862.

It is intended to prepare for publication the Medical and Surgical History of the Rebellion.

The medical portion of this work has been committed to Assistant Surgeon J. J. Woodward, United States Army, and the surgical part to Brigade-Surgeon John H. Brinton, United States Volunteers.

All medical officers are therefore requested to coöperate in this undertaking by forwarding to this office such sanitary, topographical, medical, and surgical reports, details of cases, essays, and results of investigations and inquiries as may be of value for this work, for which full credit will be given in the forthcoming volumes.

Authority has been given to both the above-named gentlemen to issue, from time to time, such circulars as may be necessary to elicit the desired facts, and the medical officers are desired to comply with the requests which may thus be made of them.

It is scarcely necessary to remind the medical officers of the Regular and Volunteer services that through the means in question much may be done to advance the science which we all have so much at heart, and to establish landmarks which will serve to guide us in future.

It is therefore confidently expected that no one will neglect this opportunity of advancing the honor of the service, the cause of humanity, and his own reputation.

WILLIAM A. HAMMOND,
Surgeon-General, U. S. Army.

CIRCULAR NO. 6.

Surgeon-General's Office,
Washington, D.C., *July* 14, 1862.

Medical Officers in charge of Military Hospitals in Washington, Baltimore, Philadelphia, and New York, and in the vicinity of those cities, will, immediately after the receipt of this order, make a special and careful examination of all convalescents under their charge, and cause all who are fit for duty to be returned at once to their regiments.

Medical Directors will be held responsible for the prompt execution of this order in their respective districts or departments.

The Army of the Potomac requires the service of all its soldiers who are able to do duty.

WILLIAM A. HAMMOND,
Surgeon-General, U. S. Army.

CIRCULAR NO. 7.

Surgeon-General's Office,
Washington, D.C., *July* 14, 1862.

In order to give greater utility to the acts of Miss D. L. Dix as "Superintendent of Women Nurses" in General Hospitals, and to make the employment of such nurses conform more closely to existing laws and orders of the War Department, the following announcement is made for the information and guidance of Medical Officers and of all concerned:

Miss Dix has been entrusted by the War Department with the duty of selecting women nurses and assigning them to general or permanent Military Hospitals. Women nurses are not to be employed in such hospitals without her sanction and approval, except in cases of urgent need.

Women nurses will be under the control and direction of the

Medical Officer in charge of the hospital to which they are assigned, and may be discharged by him if incompetent, insubordinate, or otherwise unfit for their vocation.

Miss Dix is charged with the diligent oversight of women nurses, and with the duty of ascertaining, by personal inspection, whether or not they are properly performing their duties. Medical Officers are enjoined to receive her suggestions and counsels with respect, and to carry them into effect if compatible with the hospital service.

As it will be impossible for Miss Dix to supervise in person all the Military Hospitals, she is authorized to delegate her authority, as herein defined, to subordinate agents, not to exceed one for each ci y or military district.

Women wishing employment as nurses must apply to Miss Dix, or to her authorized agents.

The Army Regulations allow one nurse to every ten patients (beds) in a General Hospital. As it is the expressed will of the Government that a portion of those nurses shall be women, and as Congress has given to the Surgeon-General authority to decide in what numbers women shall be substituted for men, it is ordered that there shall be one woman nurse to two men nurses. Medical Officers are hereby required to organize their respective hospitals accordingly.

Medical Officers requiring women nurses will apply to Miss Dix or to her authorized agent for the place where their hospitals are located.

Sisters of Charity will be employed, as at present, under special instructions from this office.

William A. Hammond,
Surgeon-General, U. S. Army.

CIRCULAR NO. 8.

Washington, *July* 24, 1862.

No candidate for service in the Women's Department for nursing in the Military Hospitals of the United States, will be received below the age of thirty-five years, nor above fifty.

Only women of strong health, not subjects of chronic disease, nor liable to sudden illnesses, need apply. The duties of the station make large and continued demands on strength.

Matronly persons of experience, good conduct, or superior education and serious disposition, will always have preference; habits of neatness, order, sobriety, and industry are prerequisites.

All applicants must present certificates of qualification and good character from at least two persons of trust, testifying to morality, integrity, seriousness, and capacity for care of the sick.

Obedience to rules of the service, and conformity to special regulations, will be required and enforced.

Compensation, as regulated by Act of Congress, forty cents a day and subsistence. Transportation furnished to and from the place of service.

Amount of luggage limited within small compass.

Dress plain (colors brown, grey, or black), and, while connected with the service, without ornaments of any sort.

No applicants accepted for less than three months' service; those for longer periods always have preference.

D. L. DIX.

Approved:

WILLIAM A. HAMMOND,
Surgeon-General.

CIRCULAR NO. 9.

Much negligence having hitherto prevailed with regard to the quarterly reports of sick and wounded, and the accompanying sanitary letter, it is hereby ordered—

I.—That all medical officers in charge of regiments or detachments of troops or of general or other hospitals, transmit forthwith to this office their quarterly reports for the quarter ending June 30, 1862.

II.—That all such officers diligently inquire whether the reports and sanitary letters of their command, for former quarters of the year commencing July 1, 1861, and ending June 30, 1862, have been duly forwarded to this office, and where this duty has been omitted, that they make out, if possible, such quarterly reports for the omitted quarters, from the records in their possession. *Where the records are incomplete*, letters will be written similar to that called for in the following paragraph:

III.—Each regimental surgeon of volunteers will prepare and forward to this office, as soon as practicable, a letter containing a brief summary of the medical history of his regiment from the time it was mustered into the service of the United States to the close of the year ending June 30, 1862.

This letter will contain the following information, viz.: (1.) A brief summary of the movements of the regiment, with sanitary descriptions of the several camp sites occupied, especially of those occupied for any considerable time; (2.) Remarks on the condition of the regiment as to food and clothing during the period; (3.) A brief sketch of the epidemics, if any, from which it may have suffered, with an outline of the symptoms, and of the treatment found most useful; (4.) A statement, from the regimental books, of the original strength of the regiment; the number of recruits who have since joined; the number of deaths from wounds and from disease; the number of discharges from service for disability; and the actual strength of the regiment on June 30, 1862, in the following form:

Regiment.	For duty.	On sick report.	In general hospital.	On furlough.	Other absentees.	TOTAL.

Any other facts may be added which are regarded as of value in the preparation of the medical and surgical history of the war.

IV.—Each Medical Officer in charge of a *hospital*, beside supplying from the hospital records all omitted quarterly reports, as directed in paragraphs I. and II., will prepare and forward to this office, as soon as possible, a letter containing the following information, viz.: (1.) The date at which the hospital was organized, by whom, and by whose order; (2.) Its location and a sanitary description of its site and surroundings; (3.) A description of the building and its several internal arrangements, accompanied by plans to make the description intelligible; (4.) Remarks on the fitness of the building for hospital purposes and the advantages and disadvantages of the plan; (5.) An account of any epidemic diseases which may have been treated in the hospital, with an outline of the symptoms and of the treatment resorted to, and of the appearances disclosed at post-mortem examinations, when held; (6.) A tabular statement of the surgical operations performed in the hospital, the injuries rendering them necessary, and the results, with any accounts of cases or other matters which may be deemed valuable contributions to the medical and surgical history of the war.

V.—It is hoped that Medical Officers will exert themselves to supply the information above called for as speedily as possible, and thus contribute their share to supply the existing deficiencies and to facilitate the collection of necessary information by the Department.

WILLIAM A. HAMMOND,
Surgeon-General, U. S. Army.

CIRCULAR NO. 10.

Surgeon-General's Office,
August 25, 1862.

I.—Immediately upon receipt of this circular, the Medical Officers of the Regular Army, and the Surgeons and Assistant Surgeons of Volunteers, will report by letter to this office their stations, or the duties to which they are assigned, and hereafter will report promptly any orders involving change of station, reporting the date of their departure and that of their arrival at their new station.

Upon the last of every month a similar report will be made.

II.—The Surgeon-General directs that official letters addressed to him by Medical Officers of the Army be written on letter paper (quarto post); also, that the letter be folded in three equal folds, parallel with the writing, and endorsed on that fold which corresponds with the top of the sheet—1st, with the name of place where written, and date; 2d, name and rank of writer; and 3d, analysis of contents.

All official communications relating to the business of the Medical Inspector's Department will be sent, under cover, to the Surgeon-General, marked on the cover "Medical Inspector's Department."

III.—In accordance with a recent Act of Congress, the Corps of Brigade Surgeons becomes the Corps of Surgeons and Assistant-Surgeons of Volunteers. The official designation and signature of these officers hereafter will be "Surgeons or Assistant-Surgeons of Volunteers," as the case may be.

IV.—Hereafter copies of all contracts made with physicians by Medical Directors or others will be immediately sent to this office.

All physicians employed on contract by the Medical Department will provide their own surgical instruments. Such instruments may be procured from Medical Purveyors, their value being deducted from the pay of the physician procuring them within the first three months after contract. The Medical Purveyors issuing instruments to contract physicians will immediately notify this office of the fact, and the money value of the instruments furnished.

V.—Physicians employed on contract will be paid on duplicate accounts in the usual form, certified to by the Medical Director, commanding officer, or surgeon in charge of hospital where service charged for was performed. These accounts will be sent to this office for approval, from whence they will be sent to the Treasury Department, by which certificates of indebtedness will be issued on which Medical Purveyors or other disbursing officers are authorized to pay. Officers certifying to such accounts will state whether or no the services were performed in the field, and whether the instruments were duly provided.

VI.—Civil nurses employed on contract will be paid by Medical Purveyors on rolls certified to by Surgeons in charge of hospitals or Medical Directors. Their pay will be $20.50 per month, and they will receive one ration per day, and the same allowance of clothing as a private soldier of infantry. Two dollars of their pay per month will be retained until the expiration of their term of service; the fact of such money having been retained being endorsed on the back of the contract. Their clothing will be issued to them by Medical Officers—the clothing account being kept in the manner prescribed by regulations for the soldier. On the contract shall be endorsed all facts ordinarily endorsed upon the descriptive list of a soldier.

VII.—Acting Medical Cadets will in no instance be mustered or paid as contract nurses. The attention of all Medical Officers employing Acting Medical Cadets is called to this prohibition of a practice fraudulent in itself, and degrading to the office of the Medical Cadet.

VIII.—The want of printed blanks is no valid excuse for not making Requisitions, Returns, and Reports required by Regulations. When there are no printed blanks, the style, classification, order, and nomenclature of the Supply Table, and of the prescribed forms, will be observed. Copies of Medical Regulations and printed blanks for Requisitions, Returns, and Reports of Sick and Wounded, may be procured by application to the Medical Director; Hospital Rolls and Certificates of Disability for Discharge, by application to the Surgeon-General.

IX.—Many Medical Officers, both regular and volunteers, have partially disregarded previous circulars issued from this office. These circulars are explanatory orders, and, in future, officers neglecting to comply with their directions will be proceeded against for disobedience of orders.

WILLIAM A. HAMMOND,
Surgeon-General, U. S. Army.

CIRCULAR No. 11.

Surgeon-General's Office,
Washington, *August* 5, 1862.

The attention of Medical Directors, and officers under their control, is called to the following requirements in relation to contracts with private physicians and their accounts, in which great irregularity exists at present:

1st. Contracts with private physicians should mention whether the service is to be rendered at a post or hospital, or in the field; or they may be made to include both hospital and field service, the sum per month agreed to be paid for each kind of service being distinctly stated. If at a post, the rate of monthly pay should be regulated by the strength of the command; if at a hospital, by the number of sick; and in neither case should it exceed $100. In the field, it should not exceed $125. (See Paragraphs 1268 and 1269, Revised Regulations, and Paragraph 1, General Order, No. 65, Adjutant-General's Office, June 12, 1862.)

2d. Every contract should be so made that it cannot be terminated by the private physician contracting, within a period of less than three months from the date of contract.

3d. A duplicate of every contract as soon as executed, should be forwarded to this Office.

4th. In cases where the services have been rendered in the field, the certificate appended to the account should state that fact, otherwise the increased allowance for field service cannot be paid.

5th. All accounts for service should be in duplicate, and should be certified by the Commanding Officer of the force with which the physician is serving, or the Surgeon in charge of the hospital, and approved by the Medical Director of the Division, Army Corps, Army, or Department.

6th. The signature of the certifying officer should be placed immediately below the certificate, and not, as now frequently occurs, in some other part of the account, thus leaving the certificate unsigned.

WILLIAM A. HAMMOND,
Surgeon-General, U. S. Army.

CIRCULAR No. 18.

Surgeon-General's Office,
Washington, *December* 5, 1862.

I.—The attention of Medical Directors is called to the numerous cases of neglect in the transmission of the Weekly Report of Hospitals, and the Monthly Report of Sick and Wounded.

In future they will require medical officers in charge of hospitals to forward to their office the Weekly Hospital Report, on the last day of each week; and they will promptly forward them to this Office, accompanied by a list of such officers as have neglected this duty.

They will also require the Monthly Report of Sick and Wounded to be forwarded to them, and will transmit them to this Office, duly filled up, as to date and place, and also accompanied by a list of names of those officers who may have failed to forward these required reports.

Medical Directors will see that the Surgeons under their direction are kept duly supplied with blank forms necessary for the above reports.

II.—Medical Directors having supervision of several General Hospitals, will require from the Surgeon in charge of each hospital a daily report of such changes as may have taken place during the preceding day. This report will state the name, company, and regiment of each soldier admitted, returned to duty, discharged, transferred to other hospitals, died, etc., etc., and these names will, from time to time, be recorded in a book kept for that purpose in the office of the Medical Director.

Every facility will be afforded the agents of the Sanitary Commission, and the friends of sick and wounded soldiers, in procuring such information concerning the inmates of hospitals, as they may, from time to time, desire.

III.—Surgeons in charge of General Hospitals will, upon receipt of this circular, report to the commanders of companies the names of any soldiers of their company deceased, or discharged from the service, while in their hospital, and concerning whom these reports have not been duly made.

These Reports will strictly conform to paragraphs 152 and 170, General Regulations, to which, for the future, particular attention must be paid.

IV.—Persons detailed for duty in any capacity in General Hospitals, by Medical Officers in charge, without proper authority, will not be recognized at this Office as hospital employés, and

Medical Officers so employing them will be personally responsible for the wages due them.

They will also be held pecuniarily responsible for any payment over their signature made to cooks and laundresses in excess of the number authorized by Regulations to the hospital under their charge.

V.—Medical Officers are explicitly informed that Regulations on the above subjects have been written and published to be observed by them, and the various infractions which, from time to time, they have allowed themselves to make, have not been overlooked in the past, nor will be for the future.

WILLIAM A. HAMMOND,
Surgeon General, U. S. Army.

CIRCULAR No. 1.

Surgeon-General's Office,
Washington, *January* 14, 1863.

By order of the War Department, the following instructions are promulgated in reference to discharges from General Hospitals:

I. Under no circumstances has the Surgeon in charge of General Hospitals, as commanding officer thereof, authority to discharge soldiers.

The final statements, and all the discharge papers, will be made out under the supervision of the military commander, and signed by him. (Vide paragraph 3 of General Orders, No. 36, of 1862.)

To prevent confusion and misunderstanding hereafter, Medical Officers in charge of General Hospitals are enjoined to be strictly guided by the above instructions.

II. Surgeons in charge of General Hospitals will, as soon as possible after the close of each month, transmit to this Office a copy of the "Statement of the Hospital Fund." (Vide paragraph 1264, General Regulations.)

Medical Directors will urge upon the Surgeons under their control the importance of prompt obedience to this regulation.

WILLIAM A. HAMMOND,
Surgeon-General, U. S. Army.

CIRCULAR No. 2.

Surgeon-General's Office,
Washington, *January* 28, 1863.

I.—By order of the War Department, the first sentence of paragraph 3, General Orders, No. 36, is modified to read as follows: "The final statements and all the discharge papers will be made out under the supervision of the Military Commander, and signed by him, when the soldier is not in a U. S. hospital or under the charge of a U. S. Surgeon. But if he is under a U. S. Surgeon or in a U. S. hospital, the Surgeon will, in either case, make out and sign the discharge and final statements, after the Military Commander has endorsed the authority to discharge the soldier upon the usual certificates of disability."

II.—Paragraph I, Circular No. 1, of 1863, from this office, is revoked, in consequence of the foregoing modification.

WILLIAM A. HAMMOND,
Surgeon-General.

CIRCULAR No. 3.

Surgeon-General's Office,
Washington, *January* 30, 1863.

I.—In consequence of the great and improper latitude which many Surgeons have allowed themselves in the administration of the Hospital Fund, the following instructions are issued defining the articles for which and for which alone the hospital fund may be expended:

The hospital fund may be expended for the purchase of—

1st. Food, solid or fluid, to be used for the diet of the sick, and not furnished by the Commissary Department or Medical Department.

2d. Articles to be used in either the preparation or serving of the food, embracing principally cooking utensils and table furniture, and not furnished by the Quartermaster's Department or Medical Department.

3d. Gas, oil, and other means of illumination, to be bought instead of candles, which are part of the soldier's ration.

Experiment has been carefully and thoroughly made in a number of our best regulated hospitals, as to the capacity of the hospital fund to support a proper diet table for the sick.

Reports from these hospitals are unanimous in the testimony that the cost of supplying such a diet exceeds the value of the hospital ration, and hence all expenditures for objects of less importance than a liberal diet are acts of injustice to the sick soldier.

II.—Upon the receipt of this circular, a return will be made to this Office, by Surgeons in charge of hospitals, of all articles of a nature not immediately perishable which have been purchased from the hospital fund, and which are now in use in the hospitals under their charge.

This return will be made in a form similar to the returns of hospital furniture now required, and will be made hereafter quarterly, upon the last day of March, June, September, and December.

Medical officers will be required to account strictly to this Department for all such articles as may be purchased from the hospital fund.

The accompanying circular, received from the Commissary General of Subsistence, is furnished for the information and guidance of Medical officers.

WILLIAM A. HAMMOND,
Surgeon-General.

* CIRCULAR.

Office Commissary General of Subsistence,
Washington, *March* 1, 1863.

HOSPITAL FUND.

HOW CREATED.

The sick in hospital not needing full rations for their subsistence, only such parts thereof are issued as are actually required for the support of themselves and authorized attendants. The difference between the number of rations due a hospital, at cost price of a complete ration at the station, and the value of the stores issued to it, during the same period and at the same prices, constitute *a credit* with the Subsistence Department in favor of the hospital. This credit is called "Hospital Fund."

ITS USES.

The Commissary who issues to a hospital is authorized to purchase for it, on the requisition of the medical officer in charge and in amount not exceeding the hospital credit at the time, as follows:

1st. Food, solid or fluid, to be used for the diet of the sick, and not furnished by the Subsistence Department or Medical Department.

2d. Articles to be used in either the preparation or serving of the food, embracing principally cooking utensils and table furniture, and not furnished by the Quartermaster's Department or Medical Department.

3d. Gas, oil, and other means of illumination, to be used instead of candles, which are part of the soldier's ration.

The Hospital Fund being thus a means for supplying the suffering sick with wants and conveniences needful for their health and more comfortable condition, not otherwise to be obtained, its manag ment should be held as a sacred trust, and its expenditure confined strictly to the purposes which this fund is designed to accomplish. Medical and hospital supplies, quartermaster's supplies, and all objects of expenditure from the appropriations of the different departments of the military service, *are not proper charges against the hospital credit.*

ITS EXPENDITURE.

The articles purchased by the Commissary for the sick in hospital are paid for out of the subsistence funds in his hands for public disbursement, on a voucher certified to by the medical officer in charge; and the hospital credit is diminished in consequence thereof by the amount of the purchases made. An expenditure of money by the Commissary for the subsistence or convenience

* This Circular is a reprint of the one on the same subject by the Commissary General, dated January 1, 1863, with slight modifications and some additional matter.

of the sick in hospital, is accounted for in the manner prescribed for other disbursements of the Subsistence Department. At large Depôts or General Hospitals, this fund may be partly expended for the benefit of the sick at dependent posts or in detachments, on requisitions approved by the Medical Director or senior Surgeon of the District.

HOW ASCERTAINED.

A "Statement of the Hospital Fund" is made out at the end of each calendar month, and appears as a part of the Commissary's "Abstract of Issues to Hospital" for that month. On it are entered the balance of credit (if any) to hospital at the end of the preceding month, and the number of rations due it in the month, at cost price; also, the stores which have been issued by the Commissary to the hospital and articles purchased by him for the sick, during this period, with the cost of each set opposite. The difference between these two amounts—credits and debits—leaves an ascertained balance of credit (if the Hospital Fund for the month has not been entirely used up), applicable to authorized expenditures for the subsistence or convenience of the sick in hospital during the following mouth. This statement may be prepared in the same manner, at any day, should there be occasion for ascertaining the exact state of the credit of a hospital at any particular date. An "Abstract of Issues to Hospital" and a "Statement of the Hospital Fund," should be made out monthly for each *separate* hospital.

HOW TRANSFERRED.

At the request of the Surgeon-General and on instructions from the Commissary General of Subsistence, Hospital Fund may be transferred as follows:

The Commissary directed to transfer any portion of this credit from a hospital he supplies to another one, drops the amount specified from his next Statement of its Hospital Fund as transferred to the hospital designated in the instructions, giving (when informed) the rank, name, regiment, or corps, and station of the Commissary who issues to it. The Commissary directed to receive a stated amount of this credit, takes up the same in favor of the designated hospital supplied by him, on his next Statement of its Hospital Fund, and as received from the one mentioned in the instructions, giving (when informed), the rank, name, regiment, or corps, and station of the Commissary who issues to such hospital.

When an officer is relieved from subsistence duty, he will give his successor a certified statement of the hospital credit of each *separate* hospital supplied by him, and will note such action on the Hospital Abstract. His successor will take up these credits in favor of each separate hospital he issues to, in manner as above explained. Hospital Fund being *a credit* only, cannot be transferred from one officer's papers to another's *as money*.

MEDICAL AND HOSPITAL SUPPLIES.

BY WHAT DEPARTMENT FURNISHED.

They are furnished *by the Medical Department* in manner and quantity as prescribed by the Regulations for that Department.

* THEIR CLASSIFICATION AND NOMENCLATURE.

HOSPITAL STORES.

Barley, in tins.
Beef, extract of.
Candles, sperm or composition.
Cinnamon, powdered.
Cocoa or chocolate.
Coffee, extract of.
Corn Starch.
Farina.
Gelatine, shred.
Ginger, powdered.
Milk, concentrated.
Nutmegs.
Pepper, black, ground.
Porter.
Sugar, white, crushed, kiln-dried.
Tea, black.
Tapioca.

STATIONERY, ETC.

Blank bks, cap, half-bound, 4 qrs.
Case book.
Envelopes, printed.
Ink.
Inkstands.
  Travelling.
Meteorological Register.
Morning Report Book.
Mucilage.
Order and Letter Book.
Prescription Book, Hospital.
  Ward, (blank, 4 quires.)
Register of Patients.
Regulations, Army.
  Medical Department.
Paper, filtering, round, gray, 10 inches.
  wrapping, white and blue.
  writing.
Pens, steel.
Penholders.
Pencils, lead, Faber's, No. 2.
Portfolio, cap size.
Sealing wax.

BEDDING.

Bed sacks.
Beds, water, of India rubber.
Blankets.
Blanket cases, canvas.
Counterpanes.
Cushions, rubber, for air or water.
  for air or water, small.
Gutta-percha bed covers.
Mattresses, hair.
  of straw, moss, or shucks.
Mosquito bars.
Pillows, hair.
Pillow cases, cotton, colored.
  linen, white.
Sheets, linen.

---

* The classifications, *Materia Medica, Instruments, Dressings, Books,* and the articles enumerated under them, are omitted here. For a *full* list of articles furnished by the Medical Department as "medical and hospital supplies," see its Standard Supply Table in Circular No. 12, of October 20, 1862, from the Surgeon-General's Office.

Hospital Clothing.

Caps.
Drawers.
Gowns, dressing.
Shirts, cotton.
Slippers.
Socks, woollen.

Furniture and Appliances.

Class No. 1.

Basins, tin, small, for dressers.
  wash, hand.
Bed pans, delf, shovel shape.
Bedsteads, iron.
Bowls, delf.
Brooms.
Brushes, scrubbing.
Buckets, leather.
  wooden.
Candlesticks.
Caldrons, with tin covers, 20 gallons.
Cleavers.
Clothes line.
Close-stools.
Corks, assorted.
Corkscrews.
Dippers, tin.
Dishes, assorted sizes.
Feeding cups, or sick feeders.
Flesh forks.
Funnels, glass.
  tin.
Graters.
Hatchet.
Hone.
Knives and Forks.
  carving.
  butchers'.
  bread.
Lanterns, glass.
Measures, graduated, glass, 4 oz.
  minim.
  tin, gallon to pint.
Medicine panniers, furnished by the list.
  measuring glasses.
  spoons, delf.
Mess chest, furnished by list.
Mills, coffee.
Mortars and pestles.
Mugs, delf.
Pill boxes, turned wood.
  machine.
  tiles.
Pitchers, delf.
Plates, delf.
Pots, chamber, delf.
  inodorous, Army pattern.
  tea, delf.
  coffee, tin.
Rain gauge.
Range, size as required, with fixtures complete.
Razor and strop, in case.
Retort, delf.
Scales and weights, prescription.
  shop.
Sheepskins, dressed for plasters.
Slates.
Spatulas.
Spirit lamp.
Spoons, table.
  tea.
Spit mugs, without tops.
Spittoons.
Steel.
Stoves, cooking, size as needed, with fixtures complete.
Test tubes.
Thermometer and Hygrometer.
Thermometer
Tin warmer, for stomach, to hold hot water.
  for feet.
Tubs, bath.
Tumblers, glass.
Urinals, glass.
Vials.
Wood-saws.

* *Class No.* 2.

Bed-ticket Frames.
Chairs.
Clocks, wooden, small.
Gridirons.
Kettles, tea, iron.
Ladles.
Looking-glasses, small.
Pans, frying.
 sauce.
Pans, tin.
Pots, mustard.
 pepper.
Refrigerators.
Sadirons.
Salt-cellars.
Tables, bedside.
Trays, butlers'.

If the expenditure of Hospital Fund be confined to the purposes indicated herein as *proper* objects for its application, (see "ITS USES," page 1,) it is believed that this credit will be ample for supplying the sick in hospital with as generous *a diet* as their several conditions may require.

J. P. TAYLOR,
Commissary General of Subsistence.

N. B.—The Hospital Fund *is not to be expended* for the following objects, Congress having therefor appropriated specific sums of money, viz:

Army medical museum; medicines and medical attendance for negro refugees, (commonly called contrabands;) and for the following objects for the regular army and volunteers, viz:

Medicines, instruments, dressings, and so forth; hospital stores, bedding, and so forth; *hospital furniture* and field equipments; medical books, stationery, *and printing;* private physicians, and medicines furnished by them; hire of clerks and laborers in purveying depots; continuing meteorological observations and tabulating the same; compensation of soldiers acting as cooks and nurses; citizen nurses; hospital clothing; care of sick soldiers in private hospitals; artificial limbs for soldiers and seamen. (See *General Orders, No.* 40, *War Department, Adjutant-General's Office, February* 11, 1863, *pages* 6, 7, *and* 8.)

CIRCULAR NO. 4.

Surgeon-General's Office,
Washington, D.C., *March* 25, 1863.

In order that the wounded may receive prompt and skilful attention during and immediately after a battle, the following instructions, compiled in part from a circular issued by the Chief Medical Director of the Army of the Potomac, October 30, 1862,

* Articles in this class are furnished by the Medical Department, "on 'requisitions for outfits,' but not on 'requisitions to replenish supplies,' unless the medical officer certifies that they cannot be purchased with the hospital fund." (See *Circular* No. 12, *of October* 20, 1862, *from the Surgeon-General's Office.*)

are published for the information and guidance of Medical Officers:

1. Before a battle, the Chief Medical Director, and the Medical Directors of Army Corps, will consult and coöperate with the officers of the Quartermaster's Department in making the necessary arrangements for the transportation of the wounded, and in instructing the drivers and assistants in the service of the ambulances and litters.

2. The Chief Medical Director will have the general superintendence of the whole ambulance and hospital service, and will give such orders for the removal, accommodation, and surgical treatment of the wounded as may be necessary. After a battle, he will cause the wounded to be removed to the permanent general hospitals, as soon as it is proper to do so, and no wounded man will be sent away from a field hospital without his authority.

3. As soon as practicable after a battle, the Chief Medical Director will transmit to the Surgeon-General a report of the action, describing the nature of the battle, the numbers engaged, the character and range of the enemy's fire, and the period and mode of removal of the wounded. He will state the number and location of the Division Hospitals, their organization and supplies, and also whether the wounded were promptly provided with food and blankets. He will transmit with this report a consolidated tabular statement of wounds received and operations performed. (See tabular statements, monthly report of sick and wounded.) Should deaths occur from anæsthetics, they will be reported in detail.

4. Medical Directors of Army Corps will apply to their Commanders, on the eve of a battle, for the necessary guards, and men for fatigue duty. These guards will be particularly careful that no stragglers be allowed about the field hospitals, using the food and comforts prepared for the wounded.

5. Previous to an engagement, each Medical Director of an Army Corps will detail a proper number of Medical Officers to remain and take care of the wounded, should a retreat be necessary. This detail he will request the Corps Commander to announce in orders.

6. Medical Directors of Army Corps, acting under the orders of the Chief Medical Director, will exercise a general superintendence over, and direction of, the medical service of their respective corps. They will establish Division Field Hospitals in the most convenient and secure positions, with ready access to water and fuel, and in buildings, where suitable ones can be obtained.

7. Medical Directors of Corps will see that the Division Hospitals are properly organized and provided with the necessary medicines, instruments, stores, and furniture.

8. They will see that the ambulances which follow the troops to succor the wounded and remove them from the field, have the necessary attendants, litters, and litter bearers, so that soldiers may have no excuse to leave the ranks for that object.

9. The Surgeon-in-Chief of each Division will exercise general supervision, under the Medical Director of the Corps, over the medical service in his Division. He will see that the officers and attendants are faithful and efficient in the discharge of their duties in the hospital, and upon the field, and that the wounded are removed from the field carefully, and with dispatch.

10. He will organize the Division Hospital, as follows:

1st. A Surgeon in charge; one Assistant-Surgeon to provide food, fuel, and water, and one Assistant-Surgeon to keep the records.

2d. Three Medical Officers, to constitute the operating staff of the hospital; three Medical Officers as assistants to each of these officers.

3d. Additional Medical Officers, Hospital Stewards, Cooks, and Nurses of the Division.

11. The Surgeon in charge will have the general superintendence, and be responsible to the Division-Surgeon for the administration of the hospital. It will be his duty to have the hospital tents properly pitched, and when houses are used, to have them put in proper order for the reception of wounded. He is to provide the necessary medical and hospital supplies, operating tables, straw or hay for bedding, blankets, and rations.

12. The Assistant-Surgeons, who are under the immediate orders of the Surgeon in charge, will aid that officer in preparing the hospital for the reception of the wounded. That duty performed, one Assistant-Surgeon will organize and take charge of a kitchen, using for this purpose the hospital mess chests, and the kettles, tins, etc., in the ambulances. The supplies of beef-extract and bread in the ambulances, and of extract of coffee, tea, condensed milk, and other hospital stores in the hospital supply wagons, will enable him to prepare quickly a sufficient quantity of palatable and nourishing food to meet the demands, until fresh beef and other subsistence stores can be provided. All the Cooks, and such of the Hospital Stewards and Nurses as may be necessary, will be placed under the orders of this Assistant-Surgeon.

13. The other Assistant-Surgeon will keep a complete record of every case brought to the hospital, giving the name, rank, company, and regiment; the seat and character of injury; the treatment; the operation, if any be performed; the name of the operator, and the result. This record will be transmitted by the Division-Surgeon to the Medical Director of the Corps, and by him sent to the Chief Medical Director.

14. This Assistant-Surgeon will make out two "Tabular statements of wounded," one of which the Division-Surgeon will transmit, within forty-eight hours after a battle, to the Chief Medical Director, and the other to the Medical Director of the Corps.

15. He will also see to the proper interment of those who die, and that each grave is marked with a headboard, with the name, rank, company, and regiment legibly inscribed upon it.

16. The three Medical Officers composing the operating staff will be selected by the Division-Surgeon, without regard to rank, but solely on account of their known prudence, judgment, and skill. The immediate responsibility of the performance of all important operations will rest with them. In all doubtful cases they will consult together, and a majority of them shall decide upon the expediency and character of the operation.

17. Each of these officers will have the aid of three Medical Officers, who, acting under his orders, will assist him in his operations.

18. The remaining Medical Officers of the Division, except one to each regiment, will be ordered to the hospitals to act as dressers and assistants generally. Those who follow the regiments to the field will establish themselves, each one at a temporary depôt, at such a distance or situation in the rear of his regiment as will insure safety to the wounded, where they will give such aid as is immeniately required; and they are here reminded that, whilst no personal consideration should interfere with their duty to the wounded, the grave responsibilities resting upon them render any unnecessary exposure improper.

19. The Division-Surgeon will order to the hospital, as soon as it is located, all the hospital supply wagons, hospital tents and furniture, and all the Hospital Stewards, Cooks, and Nurses belonging to the Division. He will notify the officer commanding the division ambulances of the position of the hospital. When his duties permit, he will give his professional services at the hospital.

20. No Medical Officer will leave the position to which he has been assigned without permission; and any officer so doing is to be reported to the Medical Director of the Corps, and to the Chief Medical Director.

21. Medical Directors of Corps, and Division-Surgeons, are required to have the following articles carried in the box of each ambulance, under the driver's seat:

Beef, extract, in 2-lb. tins,	lbs. 6.
Buckets, leather,	No. 1.
Kettles, camp,	No. 1.
Lantern and candle,	No. 1.
Spoons, table,	No. 6.
Tumblers, tin,	No. 6.
Hard bread,	lbs. 10.

The boxes will be kept locked. The Surgeon in charge of the Brigade will keep the keys, and by weekly inspections ascertain that each ambulance has its full supply. In addition to the above, each ambulance is to be furnished with two litters, and one keg filled with water.

William A. Hammond,
Surgeon-General, U. S. Army.

CIRCULAR NO. 5.

Surgeon-General's Office, *April* 13, 1863.

"The senior medical officer of hospitals, regiments, posts, or detached commands will make their requisitions for medical and hospital supplies upon the Medical Director under whom they may be serving. The Medical Director will approve or modify the requisition at his discretion, and, in ordinary cases, will transmit them to the nearest Purveyor or Medical Storekeeper, with his order for the supplies." (*Vide paragraph* 5, *Supply Table.*)

It is observed that many Surgeons have, apparently, mistaken the aims and ends of the Sanitary Commission, and the proper method of obtaining medical supplies.

Surgeons are directed, in ordinary cases, to look to no other source of supply than above indicated. Requisitions, unless otherwise specifically directed, will be made quarterly; and Surgeons who, by neglecting to make their regular requisitions, permit their hospital supplies to become exhausted, will be held strictly accountable. Special requisitions are not intended to take the place of the regular quarterly requisition. They are only permissible in cases of emergency, and the face of the requisition must state the circumstances which constitute the emergency rendering such special requisition necessary.

It is not the design of the Sanitary Commission to perform the duties which belong to the officers of this Department, nor to furnish those medical stores which ordinarily are supplied by this Department when properly asked for, or when needed. Its object and aim is to be complementary to the Medical Bureau, giving its assistance whenever, from extraordinary circumstances, emergencies arise where extraordinary means of relief are needed, and ministering to the comfort of the sick and wounded soldiers by all means belonging, properly, not to the Medical Department, but to a benevolent and far-reaching organization, such as the Sanitary Commission is.

The supplies of the Sanitary Commission, then, will not be drawn upon by medical officers to meet the current expenditures of their hospitals; and medical officers who, previous to the issue of this circular, have been in the habit of asking, without necessity, for these gratuitous issues, are believed to have done so either through ignorance of the proper means of obtaining their hospital stores, or prompted by the desire to clear themselves from a responsibility to which they would be held by this Bureau for culpable negligence in the use and waste of supplies received from the regular purveying officers of the Medical Department.

The mode of obtaining supplies, detailed in the opening paragraph of this circular, will be hereafter strictly followed.

W. A. Hammond,
Surgeon-General.

CIRCULAR NO. 6.

Surgeon-General's Office,
Washington, D.C., *May* 4, 1863.

I. From the reports of Medical Inspectors and the Sanitary reports to this office, it appears that the administration of calomel has so frequently been pushed to excess by military surgeons as to call for prompt steps by this office to correct this abuse; an abuse the melancholy effects of which, as officially reported, have exhibited themselves not only in innumerable cases of profuse salivation, but in the not infrequent occurrence of mercurial gangrene.

It seeming impossible in any other manner to properly restrict the use of this powerful agent, it is directed that it be struck from the Supply Table, and that no further requisitions for this medicine be approved by Medical Directors. This is done with the more confidence as modern pathology has proved the impropriety of the use of mercury in very many of those diseases in which it was formerly unfailingly administered.

II. The records of this office having conclusively proved that diseases prevalent in the Army may be treated as efficiently without tartar emetic as therewith, and the fact of its remaining upon the Supply Table being a tacit invitation to its use, tartar emetic is also struck from the Supply Table of the Army.

No doubt can exist that more harm has resulted from the misuse of both these agents, in the treatment of disease, than benefit from their proper administration.

W. A. Hammoed,
Surgeon-General.

Directions concerning the Duties of Medical Purveyors and Medical Storekeepers, and the Manner of Obtaining and Accounting for Medical and Hospital Supplies for the Army.

STANDARD SUPPLY TABLE.

CIRCULAR NO. 7.

Surgeon-General's Office,
May 7, 1863.

DUTIES OF MEDICAL PURVEYORS AND MEDICAL STOREKEEPERS.

1. Medical Purveyors are charged, under the direction of the Surgeon-General, with the selection and purchase of all medical and hospital supplies for the Army. In all cases of emergency they may provide such additional accommodations for the sick and wounded of the Army, and may transport such medical and hospital supplies, as circumstances may render necessary. In all *cases of emergency* they shall promptly issue supplies on special requisitions made directly upon them, and such special requisitions shall consist simply of a list of the articles and quantities required, and be dated and signed by the Medical Officer who makes the requisition. The nature of the emergency must be stated, otherwise the requisition will be referred to the Medical Director.

2. Except in the "cases of emergency" referred to in the pre-

ceding paragraph, Medical Purveyors and Medical Storekeepers will issue medical and hospital supplies on the order of the Surgeon-General, the Assistant-Surgeon-General, or a Medical Director.

3. Medical Storekeepers are charged, under the direction of the Surgeon-General and Medical Purveyors, with the storing and safe-keeping of medical and hospital supplies, and with the duties of receiving, issuing, and accounting for the same, according to regulations. Medical and hospital supplies transferred to Medical Storekeepers by Medical Purveyors will be receipted for as invoiced without breaking packages, provided the number of packages correspond with the invoice, that they are in good shipping condition, and that there be no reason to suppose the contents broken or defective.

4. Medical Purveyors will be responsible for the quality of the medical and hospital supplies purchased by them, and they are directed to have surgical instruments made in the best manner, of the best materials, and according to patterns approved by the Surgeon-General. Each instrument is to be inspected, and each chain-saw tested on fresh bone by them, or under their supervision, before being paid for or issued.

5. Medical Purveyors and Medical Storekeepers will be held responsible that the medical and hospital supplies issued or transferred by them are well-packed; that each article is designated by the name of the maker or vendor, and that each package is legibly and correctly marked with the address of the officer for whom it is intended, and with its weight and contents, whether medicines, instruments, dressings, books and stationery, bedding, clothing, or furniture and appliances.

6. In issuing or transferring medical and hospital supplies, Medical Purveyors and Medical Storekeepers will furnish a packer's list and invoice to the officer who is to receive them, and transmit a duplicate of the invoice to the Surgeon-General. In turning over supplies to a Quartermaster for storage or transportation, they will forward to the Surgeon-General, with the invoice, the Quartermaster's receipt for the packages.

7. In issuing medical and hospital supplies, Medical Purveyors and Medical Storekeepers will, ordinarily, be governed by the Supply Table; but when articles are required in large quantities for use in hospitals and at permanent posts, and not for re-issue, or for field service, they will disregard the size of packages designated in that table, and will issue in such packages as they may deem most advantageous for the public service.

8. Medical Purveyors and all other disbursing officers will render direct to the Second Auditor of the Treasury, within ten days after the expiration of each successive month, a duly certified *monthly statement* of all public moneys on hand from last returns, received, disbursed, or transferred during the month, the balance remaining on hand, and where deposited (Form 1). A duplicate

of this monthly statement will be forwarded, at the same time, to the Surgeon-General, with an estimate of the funds required during the ensuing month (Form 2).

9. Medical Purveyors and all other medical disbursing officers will also render direct to the Second Auditor of the Treasury, within *one month* after the expiration of each successive quarter, a *quarterly account current* of moneys received, expended, &c., during the quarter (Form 3), with an *abstract of disbursements* (Form 4), and proper *vouchers* (Form 5). A duplicate of the account current, and of the abstract, will be forwarded at the same time to the Surgeon-General.

10. Medical Purveyors and all other medical disbursing officers will render their summary statements, accounts, abstracts, and vouchers, as above directed, when they cease to disburse, from change of duty or otherwise.

11. Medical Purveyors and Medical Storekeepers will make to the Surgeon-General, at the end of each fiscal quarter, returns in duplicate of medical and hospital property (Form 6), with an abstract of receipts and issues (Form 7), giving the number of the voucher and the name of the person from whom received and to whom issued

12. Medical Purveyors and Medical Storekeepers will give bonds in such sums as the Secretary of War may require, with security to be approved by him. Medical Officers temporarily assigned to duty as Acting Medical Purveyors are not required to give bonds.

MEDICAL AND HOSPITAL SUPPLIES.

13. The standard of medical and hospital supplies for the Army is the Supply Table. It is not the design of the Department to confine Medical Officers absolutely to that table, either in variety or quantity, but only to establish a standard for their guidance in making requisitions for supplies, leaving individual preferences to be indulged at the discretion of the Medical Directors or the Surgeon-General. Neither is it supposed that the quantities of the table will always meet the necessities of unusual emergencies, as during epidemics, or in unhealthy seasons and localities; and Medical Officers who allow their supplies to be exhausted through any such contingencies, without timely notice of their approaching necessities, will be held to a strict accountability.

14. Medical Purveyors and Medical Storekeepers at depôts for issue, and at field depôts, and the senior Medical Officers of hospitals, regiments, posts, or detached commands, will make their requisitions for medical and hospital supplies upon the Medical Director under whom they may be serving. The Medical Director will approve or modify the requisitions at his discretion; and, in ordinary cases, will transmit them to the nearest Purveyor or Medical Storekeeper, with his order for the supplies. If, however, the amount required be large, and the situation and nature of the

service permit, the Medical Director will transmit the requisitions, with his recommendations indorsed thereon, to the Surgeon-General.

15. Requisitions for medical and hospital supplies are to be made in duplicate. In preparing them, Medical Officers will conform to the Standard Supply Table, both in the articles and quantities asked for, avoiding fractions in quantities. When increased quantities or additional articles are required, satisfactory reasons must be assigned, or they will not be supplied.

16. Requisitions for outfits of medical and hospital supplies will be made for three months, and in the form of a letter, stating the number of men or beds to be supplied, and whether for general hospitals, permanent posts, or field service. If for permanent posts, the amount of hospital accommodations must be stated, so that, if less than one hundred beds, the allowance of bedding, hospital clothing, furniture, and appliances may be correspondingly reduced.

17. Requisitions to replenish medical and hospital supplies will always be made in detail, according to Form 8, and for those articles only that are really deficient in quantity. If the supplies are to be obtained from the principal purveying depôts, these requisitions will be made quarterly; if from department or field depôts, they will be made at such times and for such periods as the Medical Director may prescribe. Special requisitions are not intended to take the place of the regular quarterly requisition. They are only permissible in cases of emergency, and the face of the requisition must state the circumstances which constitute the emergency rendering such special requisition necessary.

18. When it is necessary to obtain medical and hospital supplies, and recourse cannot be had to a Medical Purveyor or Storekeeper, they may be purchased by a Quartermaster, on special requisition made according to Form 9 and Account Form 10.—(See Army Regulations, paragraph 1233.) A triplicate of all such special requisitions, giving the name and station of the officer upon whom it is made, is to be transmitted, through the Medical Director, to the Surgeon-General, for his information, and as a guide in auditing the account when presented.

19. Those articles of the Standard Supply Table which are printed in italics will be furnished only on special requisitions approved by the Surgeon-General.

20. Articles of furniture and appliances in Class No. 2 will be issued on "requisitions for outfits," but not on "requisitions to replenish supplies," unless the Medical Officer certifies that they cannot be purchased with the hospital funds.

21. Medical Officers having charge of medical and hospital supplies will make to the Surgeon-General annually, on the 31st of December, and whenever relieved therefrom, returns in duplicate (Form 6). These returns will exhibit the condition of the sup-

plies, and state to whom, or from whom, and when and where issued or received.

22. Hospital clothing belongs to the United States, and will only be worn by patients during their stay in the hospital. Each article will be marked as hospital property, and with the number of the bed for which it is appropriated.

23. An officer transferring medical and hospital supplies will furnish a certified invoice and packer's list to the officer who is to receive them, and transmit a duplicate of the invoice to the Surgeon-General. The receiving officer will furnish a receipt to the officer making the issue, with a report of the quality and condition of the articles, and transmit a duplicate of the receipt and report to the Surgeon-General. A Medical Officer who turns over medical supplies to a Quartermaster for storage or transportation will forward to the Surgeon-General, with the invoice, the Quartermaster's receipt for the packages.

24. Medical Officers will take up and account for all medical and hospital supplies of the Army that come into their possession, and report, when they know it, to whose account they are to be credited.

25. The transfer of surgical instruments issued to Medical Officers for their personal use is positively forbidden. Each Medical Officer will retain those instruments in his immediate possession so long as he remains in the Army, and will be held responsible for their complete and serviceable condition, and for their easy accessibility at all times. If the instruments be lost, destroyed, or damaged, they must be replaced or repaired as soon as possible by requisition upon the nearest Medical Purveyor, setting fully the causes of such loss or damage. If the loss or damage be from the unavoidable casualties of the service, the expense of replacing or repairing the instruments will be paid by the Medical Department; if from any other causes, such expenses must be paid by the Medical Officer.

26. When a Medical Officer leaves the Army, he will deliver his instruments to the nearest Medical Purveyor, taking receipts therefor in detail; and if transportation be required, he will take receipts for the package containing the instruments from an officer of the Quartermaster's Department.

27. Staff-Surgeons, Staff-Assistant-Surgeons, and Medical Officers in charge of General Hospitals, will be furnished with *additional instruments*, on special requisition, provided the reasons for requiring them be given and prove satisfactory to the Surgeon-General.

28. The Surgeon-General, Assistant-Surgeon-General, Medical-Inspector-General, and Medical Inspectors are allowed the same instruments as Staff-Surgeons.

29. These instruments will be accounted for to the Surgeon-General on the 31st December annually (Form 11), in which the true condition of each must be stated; and if any be lost or

damaged, a report of the facts and circumstances attending such loss or damage must be given.

30. Amputating, trephining, exsecting, general operating, and pocket instruments that do not correspond in detail with the sets prescribed by regulations, will be accounted for on the regular property returns as amputating, trephining, exsecting, general operating, and pocket sets, without designating the special instruments comprising each set, or making a special return thereof.

31. Medical officers will report to the Surgeon-General and to the issuing officer all defects observed in the quality, quantity, or packing of medical and hospital supplies, or in the material or construction of their surgical instruments, giving the name of the vendor or maker, and of the officer by whom they were issued.

32. Carbolic acid (Bower's), sulphate of iron, nitrate of lead, chlorinated lime, permanganate of potash, or charcoal, will be furnished as antiseptics or disinfectants, when required.

33. Applications for microscopes by medical officers in charge of general hospitals will be favorably considered, provided the evidence is satisfactory that the officer will use the instrument for the benefit of science, and will report the results of his observations to the Surgeon-General.

34. The dissecting case, obstetrical case, pocket case for hospitals, teeth-extracting case, medicine case, and medicine panniers, will be issued, receipted, and returned for as *sets*, without stating their contents in detail

35. No officer shall drop from his return any medical or hospital property as worn out or unserviceable until it has been condemned after proper inspection, and ordered to be so dropped. Articles purchased with the hospital fund will not be accounted for on the regular return of medical and hospital property.

36. Requisitions on officers of the Quartermaster's Department for hospitals, and the necessary fixtures and hospital tents, for fuel, straw, and wagons for the transportation of the sick and wounded, and of medical and hospital supplies, etc., will be made by the senior surgeon and approved by the commanding officer or Medical Director. Requisitions for hospitals will state the number and dimensions of the rooms required, the use to which they are severally to be applied, and the strength of the command for which they are estimated, duplicates of which will be transmitted to the Surgeon-General.

37. Surgical instruments, medicine cases, panniers, and mess chests that need and are worth repairing, or that require to be refilled, will be invoiced and sent, when circumstances permit, to the nearest Medical Purveyor or Medical Storekeeper, and are not to be submitted to inspection with a view to condemnation, unless the probable expense of transportation and repair will exceed the value of the articles.

38 All empty boxes, cans, and bottles, in which medical and hospital supplies were received, are to be carefully cleansed and

preserved from damage. Such as will not be required for further use in the hospital will be disposed of, at either private or public sale, at least once a year, and the net proceeds of such sales will be turned over to the nearest Medical Purveyor, and be receipted for by him as public funds pertaining to the Medical Department of the Army. At stations near a Medical Purveyor, these articles will be turned over to that officer.

39. In all official lists of medical supplies, the classification, order, and nomenclature of the Standard Supply Table will be strictly followed. The whole table need not be transcribed, but the names of those articles only which are accounted for or required.

STANDARD SUPPLY TABLE.

ARTICLES.	ALLOWANCE FOR THREE MONTHS— For General Hospitals.						For a Reg't or 1,000 troops.	
	100 Beds.	200 Beds.	300 Beds.	400 Beds.	500 Beds.	1,000 Beds.	At Perm'nt Posts.	In the field
MATERIA MEDICA.								
Acaciæ Pulvis, in ½ lb. bottles..............oz.	32	56	80	104	128	232	32	8
Acidum Aceticum, in ½ lb. g. s. bottles....oz.	8	16	24	32	40	72	8	....
Citricum, in ½ lb. bottles..............oz.	16	32	48	56	64	120	16	....
Muriaticum, in ½ lb. g. s. bottles.......oz.	8	8	16	16	24	40	8	....
Nitricum, in ½ lb. g. s. bottles........oz.	8	16	16	24	32	56	8	....
Phosphoricum Dilutum, in 2 oz. g. s. bottles..............................oz.	2	2	3	3	4	7	2	....
Sulphuricum, in ½ lb. g. s. bottles.....oz.	8	8	16	16	24	40	8	....
Aromaticum, in ½ lb. g. s. bottles.oz.	16	32	48	56	64	120	16	8
Tannicum, in 1 oz. bottles.............oz.	4	6	8	10	12	22	4	1
Tartaricum, in 8 oz. bottles........... oz.	32	56	80	104	128	232	32	....
Æther Fortior, in ½ lb. g. s. bottles and ½ lb. tins, soldered..........................ob.	64	112	160	208	256	464	64	32
Ætheris Spiritus Compositus, in ½ lb. g. s. bottles..............................oz.	16	32	48	56	64	120	16	16
Nitrici, in ½ lb. g. s. bottles...........oz.	48	96	144	176	208	384	48	32
Alcohol Fortius, in 32 oz bottles.... ..bottles.	24	36	48	60	72	144	24	6
Aloes Pulvis, in 2 oz. bottles...............oz.	2	4	6	6	8	14	2	....
Alumen, in ½ lb. bottles..................oz.	16	32	40	48	56	104	16	8
Ammoniæ Carbonas, in ½ lb. bottles.......oz.	16	32	40	48	64	112	16	8
Liquor, in ½ lb. g. s. bottles. ....oz.	96	164	224	288	352	640	96	32
Murias, in ½ lb. bottles...............oz.	8	16	24	32	40	72	8	...
Spiritus Aromaticus, in 4 oz. g. s. bottles..............................oz.	4	8	12	16	20	36	4	4
Argenti Nitras, in 1 oz. g. s. bottles........oz.	2	3	4	5	6	11	2	1
Fusum, in 1 oz. bottles................oz.	2	3	4	5	6	11	2	1
Arsenitis Potassæ Liquor, in 4 oz. bottles...oz.	4	8	12	16	20	36	4	...
Asafœtida, in 4 oz. bottles................oz.	4	8	12	16	16	32	4	....
Bismuthi Subcarbonas, in 2 oz. bottles......oz.	2	4	6	8	10	18	2	...
Camphora, in 8 oz. bottles ....oz.	8	16	24	32	40	72	8	8
Cantharidis Pulvis, in 2 oz. bottles.........oz.	2	2	2	4	4	8	2	....
Ceratum, in 8 oz. tins.................oz	24	40	56	72	88	160	24	8
Capsici Pulvis, in 8 oz. bottles.............oz.	8	16	24	24	32	56	8	8
Catechu, in 8 oz. bottles....................oz.	8	16	24	24	32	56	8	...
Cera Alba, in paper.........................oz.	32	32	48	48	64	112	32	4
Ceratum Adipis, in 1 lb. pots..............lb.	10	18	26	32	40	72	10	4
Resinæ, in 1 lb. pots..................lb.	2	4	5	6	8	14	2	1
Cinchonæ Calisayæ Pulvis, in ½ lb. bottles.oz.	16	24	32	40	48	88	16	....
Cinchoniæ Sulphas, in 2 oz. bottles........oz.	40	50	60	70	80	150	40	24
Chlorinium, (the materials for preparing,) in a package.............................no.	1	2	3	4	5	9	1	....
Chloroformum, in ½ lb. g. s. bottles and ½ lb. tins, soldered......................... .oz.	32	64	80	96	112	208	32	32
Collodium, in 1 oz. bottles..................oz.	2	3	4	5	6	11	2	1
Copaiba, in 1 lb. bottles...................oz.	64	96	102	128	144	272	64	16
Creasotum, in 2 oz. g. s. bottles............oz.	4	6	8	10	12	22	4	4
Creta Præparata, in ½ lb. bottles..........oz.	16	24	32	40	48	88	16	....
Cubebæ Oleo-resina. (ex. Cubebæ Fl. U. S. P., 1850,) in 8 oz. g. s. bottles...............oz.	8	16	24	32	40	72	8	....
Cupri Sulphas, in 2 oz. bottles..............oz.	2	4	6	8	10	18	2	2
Extractum Aconiti Radicis Fluidum, in ½ lb. bottles...............................oz.	8	16	24	32	40	72	8	8

STANDARD SUPPLY TABLE.

Articles.	Allowance for three months— For General Hospitals.						For a Reg't or 1,000 troops.	
	100 Beds.	200 Beds.	300 Beds.	400 Beds.	500 Beds.	1,000 Beds.	At Perm'nt Posts.	In the field.
Materia Medica.—Continued.								
Extractum Belladonnæ, in 1 oz. pots.......oz.	1	2	3	4	5	9	1	1
Buchu Fluidum, in ½ lb. bottles.......oz.	16	24	32	40	48	88	16	....
Cinchonæ Fluidum, (with aromatics,) in ½ lb. bottles.......................oz.	16	32	48	56	64	120	16	16
Colchici Seminis Fluidum, in 4 oz. bottles ....oz.	8	12	16	20	24	44	8	8
Colocynthidis Compositum, in 8 oz. pots oz.	8	16	24	32	32	64	8	8
Conii, in 1 oz. pots.....................oz.	1	2	3	4	5	9	1	....
Ergotæ Fluidum, in 2 oz. bottles.......oz.	2	4	6	8	8	16	2	....
Gentianæ Fluidum, in ½ lb bottles.....oz.	16	32	48	64	80	144	16	....
Glycyrrhizæ, in paper................oz.	64	96	128	160	192	352	64	....
Hyoscyami, in 1 oz. pots.... ....oz	1	2	3	4	5	9	1	....
Ipecacuanhæ Fluidum, in ½ lb. bottles.oz.	8	16	24	32	40	72	8	8
Nucis Vomicæ, in 1 oz. pots...........oz.	1	2	3	4	5	9	1	....
Pruni Virginianæ Fluidum, in ½ lb. bottles...............................oz.	8	16	24	32	40	72	8	....
Rhei Fluidum, in ½ lb. bottles.........oz.	8	16	24	32	40	72	8	....
Senegæ Fluidum, in ½ lb. bottles......oz.	8	16	24	32	40	72	8	8
Spigeliæ Fluidum, in ½ lb. bottles.... oz.	8	16	16	24	24	48	8	....
Valerianæ Fluidum, in ½ lb. bottles...oz	8	16	24	32	40	72	8	....
Veratri Viridis Fluidum, in 2 oz. bottles ....oz.	2	4	6	6	8	14	2	....
Zingiberis Fluidum, in ½ lb. bottles... oz.	16	24	32	40	48	88	16	16
Ferri Chloridi Tinctura, in ½ lb. g. s. bottles ....oz.	16	32	48	56	64	120	16	8
Iodidi Syrupus, in ½ lb. g. s. bottles...oz.	16	24	24	32	32	64	16	....
et Quiniæ Citras, in 1 oz. bottles.......oz.	4	6	8	10	12	22	4	1
Persulphatis Liquor, in 4 oz. g. s. bottles oz.	4	8	12	16	20	36	4	4
Pulvis, in 1 oz. g. s. bottles........oz.	1	2	3	4	5	9	1	1
Sulphas, in 4 oz. bottles...............oz.	4	4	8	8	12	20	4	....
Oxidum Hydratum, (the materials for,) in package..................... .....no.	1	1	1	1	1	2	1	....
Glycyrrhizæ Pulvis, in ½ lb. bottles.......oz.	8	16	24	32	32	64	8	....
Glycerina, (pure and inodorous,) in ½ lb. g. s. bottles.................................oz.	16	24	32	40	40	80	16	8
Hydrargyri Chloridum Corrosivum, in 1 oz. g. s. bottles..........................oz.	1	2	2	3	3	6	1	....
Iodidum Flavum, in 1 oz. bottles. .....oz	1	1	2	2	2	4	1	....
Oxidum Rubrum, in 1 oz. bottles......oz	1	1	2	2	3	4	1	....
Pilulæ, in 8 oz. pots...................oz.	8	16	24	32	40	72	8	8
Unguentum, in 1 lb. pots... ....lb.	1	2	3	4	4	8	1	1
Nitratis, in 4 oz. pots..............oz.	4	8	8	12	16	28	4	4
Iodinium, in 1 oz. g. s. bottles............oz.	4	6	6	8	8	16	4	2
Ipecacuanhæ Pulvis, in ½ lb. bottles......oz.	8	16	16	24	24	48	8	8
et Opii Pulvis, in ¼ lb. bottles.........oz.	8	16	24	32	40	72	8	8
Linum, in tins...........................lb.	6	12	18	24	30	54	6	....
Lini Pulvis, in tins.........................lb.	16	32	48	48	56	104	16	8
Magnesia, in 4 oz. bottles..................oz.	8	16	16	20	24	44	8	....
Magnesiæ Sulphas, in ½ oz. papers and 8 lb. tins...............................lbs.	16	24	32	40	48	88	16	8
Morphiæ Sulphas, in ½ oz. bottles.........oz	½	½	¾	1	1¼	2¼	½	½
Oleum Cinnamomi, in 1 oz. g. s. bottles. ..oz.	1	1	2	2	3	5	1	....

STANDARD SUPPLY TABLE.

Articles.	Allowance for three months— For General Hospitals. 100 Beds.	200 Beds.	300 Beds.	400 Beds.	500 Beds.	1,000 Beds.	For a Reg't or 1,000 troops. At Perm'nt Posts.	In the field.
Materia Medica.—Continued.								
Olei Menthæ Piperitæ Tinctura, in ½ lb bottles ....oz.	16	24	32	40	48	88	16	....
Oleum Morrhuæ, in 32 oz. bottles ....bottles.	10	15	20	25	30	55	10	....
Olivæ, in 32 oz. bottles ....bottles.	4	8	12	16	20	36	4	2
Ricini, in 32 oz. bottles ....bottles.	8	12	16	20	24	44	8	4
Oleum Terebinthinæ, in 32 oz. bottles..bottles.	2	4	6	8	10	18	2	1
Tiglii, in 1 oz. g. s. bottles ....oz.	1	1	2	2	3	5	1	1
Opii Pulvis, in ½ lb. bottles ....oz.	8	16	16	24	24	48	8	8
Tinctura, in ½ lb. bottles ....oz.	16	32	48	56	64	120	16	16
Camphorata, in ½ lb. bottles ....oz.	16	32	48	56	64	120	16	16
Pilulæ Camphoræ (gra. 2) et Opii. (gr. 1,) in g. s. bottles ....doz.	....	....	....	....	....	....	....	8
Catharticæ Compositæ, in g. s. bottles.doz.	8	16	24	32	40	72	8	8
Opii, in g. s. bottles ....doz.	....	....	...	....	....	....	....	8
Plumbi Acetas, in ½ lb. bottles ....oz.	8	16	24	32	40	72	8	8
Podophylli Resini, in 1 oz. bottles ....oz.	1	1	2	2	3	5	1	....
Potassæ Acetas, in ½ lb. bottles ....oz.	8	16	24	32	40	72	8	....
Bicarbonas, in ½ lb. bottles ....oz.	8	16	24	32	40	72	8	8
Bitartras, in ½ lb. bottles ....oz.	16	32	32	48	48	96	16	....
Chloras, in ½ lb. bottles ....oz.	16	32	32	48	48	96	16	8
Nitras, in ½ lb. bottles ....oz.	8	8	16	16	24	40	8	....
Potassii Iodidum, in ½ lb. bottles ....oz.	24	48	64	80	96	176	24	8
Quiniæ Sulphas, compressed in 5 oz. tins...oz.	20	30	40	50	60	110	20	10
Rheum ....oz.	4	4	4	8	8	16	4	....
Rhei Pulvis, in 4 oz. bottles ....oz.	4	8	12	16	16	32	4	....
Sapo, in paper ....lbs.	8	12	16	20	24	44	8	8
Scillæ Pulvis, in 1 oz. bottles ....oz.	4	4	6	6	8	14	4	2
Syrupus, in 1 lb. bottles ....lbs.	8	14	20	26	42	58	8	4
Sinapis Nigræ Pulvis, in 6 lb. tins ....lbs.	6	12	18	18	24	42	6	6
Sodæ Chlorinatæ Liquor, in 1 lb. g. s. bottles ....lbs.	6	9	12	15	15	30	6	1
Bicarbonas, in ½ lb. bottles ....oz.	16	32	40	48	56	104	16	8
Boras, in ½ lb. bottles ....oz.	8	16	16	24	24	48	8	....
et Potassæ Tartras, in ½ lb. bottles....oz.	32	64	64	80	96	176	32	16
Spiritus Lavandulæ Compositus, in ½ lb. bottles ....oz.	16	24	32	40	48	88	16	....
Frumenti, in 32 oz. bottles ....bottles.	72	120	168	216	264	480	72	24
Vini Gallici, in 32 oz. bottles ....bottles.	12	24	24	36	36	72	12	6
Sulphur, in ½ lb. bottles ....oz.	16	24	32	40	48	88	16	....
Strychnia, in ⅛ oz. bottles ....oz	⅛	⅛	¼	¼	¼	½	⅛	...
Vinum Xericum, in 32 oz. bottles .... bottles.	24	36	48	60	72	132	24	....
Zinci Acetas, in 1 oz. bottles ....oz.	2	4	5	6	7	13	2	....
Carbonas, in 1 oz. bottles ....oz.	1	2	3	4	5	9	1	....
Chloridi Liquor, in 1 lb. g. s. bottles....oz	48	80	96	112	128	240	48	16
Sulphas, in 1 oz. bottles ....oz.	2	4	5	6	7	13	2	1
Hospital Stores.								
Barley, in tins ....lbs.	10	15	20	25	30	55	10	...
Beef, extract of, in 2 lb. tins ....lbs.	24	24	36	36	48	84	24	24
Candles, Sperm or Composition, half length, in boxes ....lbs.	2	2	4	4	6	10	2	2

STANDARD SUPPLY TABLE.

ARTICLES.	ALLOWANCE FOR THREE MONTHS— For General Hospitals. 100 Beds.	200 Beds.	300 Beds.	400 Beds.	500 Beds.	1,000 Beds.	For a Reg't or 1,000 troops. At Perm'nt Posts.	In the field
HOSPITAL STORES.—Continued.								
Cinnamon, powdered, in ¼ lb. bottles.....lbs.	¼	½	¾	1	1	2	½	....
Cocoa or Chocolate, in tins or cakes.......lbs.	10	15	20	25	30	55	10	....
Coffee, extract of, in ½ gallon tins.......gals.	....	....	....	....	....	....	....	4
Corn Starch, in tins.......................lbs.	10	15	20	25	30	55	10	....
Farina, in tins............................lbs.	10	15	20	25	30	55	10	....
Gelatine, shred, in ¼ lb. packages........lbs.	1	1½	2	2½	3	5½	1	....
Ginger, powdered, in ½ lb. bottles........lbs.	½	1	1½	2	2	4	1	....
Milk, concentrated, in 1 lb. tins..........lbs.	...	...	....	....	....	....	....	16
Nutmegs, in ¼ lb. bottles.................lbs.	¼	½	¾	1	1	2	¼	¼
Pepper, black, ground, in ⅓ lb. bottles... lbs	1	1½	2	2½	3	5½	1	....
Porter, in pint bottles................bottles.	96	168	240	312	384	696	96	....
Sugar, white, crushed, kiln-dried, in boxes or tins..........lbs.	24	48	72	96	120	216	24	12
Tea, black, in tins or original chests.......lbs.	15	25	35	45	55	100	12	5
Tapioca, in tins...........................lbs.	8	12	16	20	24	44	8	...
INSTRUMENTS.								
Cupping Glasses, assorted sizes............no.	12	18	24	24	36	36	12	....
Tins ....do.................no.	12	12	18	18	24	36	12	12
Dissecting Instruments, (see list)........cases.	1	1	1	1	2	2	1	....
Lancets, thumb..........................no.	2	3	4	5	6	8	2	2
Obstetrical Case, (see list)...............case.	....	....	....	....	....	....	2	....
Pocket Case, (see list)..................cases.	1	1	2	2	3	3	1	1
Probangs.................................no.	6	6	9	9	12	18	6	6
Scarificator..............................no.	2	2	2	3	4	4	2	2
Scissors, large and small..................no.	2	2	4	4	6	8	2	2
Speculum for the ear......................no.	1	1	1	1	1	1	1	....
for the vagina, glass ....no	....	....	....	....	....	...	1	....
Spongeholder, for the throat..............no.	1	1	1	2	2	2	1	1
Stethoscope ....no.	1	1	1	1	1	1	1	....
Stomach Pump, in case....................no.	....	....	...	....	1	1	1	....
Stomach Tube............................no.	1	1	1	1	....	....	....	1
Syringe, rubber, self-injecting, No. 1.......no.	2	2	2	3	3	4	2	2
hard rubber, 8 ounce.................no.	1	1	1	1	1	2	1	....
4 ounce.................no.	....	....	....	....	....	....	....	1
universal ....no.	....	....	....	....	1	1	1	....
hypodermic, 3 points.................no.	1	1	1	1	1	1	1	....
penis, glass, in case ....no.	6	6	8	8	12	18	12	6
vagina, hard rubber, 1 } glass, 2....... } ....case.	....	....	....	....	....	....	1	....
Teeth-extracting instruments, (see list)...case.	1	1	1	1	1	1	1	1
Tongue Depressor, hinged................no.	1	1	2	2	3	4	1	1
Tourniquets, field. ....no.	....	...		....	....	...	....	8
screw, with pad.......................no.	1	1	1	2	2	2	1	2
Trusses, inguinal, double.................no.	1	1	1	1	2	2	1	...
single ... .no.	3	3	4	4	6	6	6	4
Vaccinator, (spring) ... .no.	....	....	....	....	....	1	1	1
Vaccine virus, issued as required, crusts ...no.	....	....	....	....	....	....	....	....

STANDARD SUPPLY TABLE.

Articles.	Allowance for three months— For General Hospitals						For a Reg't or 1,000 troops.	
	100 Beds.	200 Beds.	300 Beds.	400 Beds.	500 Beds.	1,000 Beds.	At Perm'nt Posts.	In the field
Dressing, etc.								
Adhesive Plaster, 5 yards in a can......yards.	10	15	20	25	35	55	10	5
Binder's Boards, 2½ by 12 inches......pieces.	6	6	12	12	18	24	6	8
4 by 17 inches.....................pieces.	6	6	12	12	18	24	6	8
Cotton Bats.............................no.	2	3	4	5	6	10	2	2
Wadding.........................sheets.	2	3	4	5	6	10	2	1
Flannel, red, all wool..................yards.	4	6	8	10	10	20	4	4
Gutta-Percha Cloth.....................yards.	4	8	12	16	20	36	4	2
Ichthyocolla Plaster, 1 yard in a case...yards.	4	6	8	8	12	20	4	5
Lint, patent, linen or flax................lbs.	4	6	8	10	12	24	4	4
picked or scraped linen..............lbs.	2	4	6	8	10	18	2	2
Muslin, bleached, unsized, 1 yard wide.yards.	20	30	40	50	60	120	20	10
Napkins for Ophthalmia....................no.	12	12	18	18	24	36	12	....
Needles 25, cotton 1 spool, thimble 1, in case....................................no.	2	2	2	2	4	4	2	1
Oakum, fine, picked......................lbs.	10	15	20	25	30	60	10	5
Oiled muslin, in 4½ yard pieces........yards.	2¼	4½	4½	6¾	9	18	2¼	2¼
Silk, in 4½ yard pieces...........yards.	2¼	4½	4½	6¾	9	18	2¼	2¼
Pencils, hair, (assorted sizes,) 12 in a vial..no.	12	24	24	36	36	48	12	12
Pins.......................................papers.	2	4	6	8	10	20	2	2
Roller Bandages, assorted, in a pasteboard box—1 doz. 1 in. by 1 yard, 2 doz. 2 in. by 3 yards, 2 doz. 2½ in. by 3 yards, 1 doz. 3 in. by 4 yards, 1 doz. 3½ in. by 5 yards, ½ doz. 4 in. by 6 yards, ½ doz. 4 in. by 8 yards.doz.	16	32	48	64	80	160	16	16
Silk, green, for shades.................yards.	1	2	2	3	3	4	1	1
saddlers', for ligatures................oz.	¼	½	¾	1	1	2	¼	¼
Splints, in one package, 6 for forearm, 4 for leg, 6 large coaptation, 4 small coaptation.................................set.	1	1	1	2	2	4	1	1
Splint's, Smith's anterior..................no.	3	4	5	6	6	12	3	3
Sponge, fine, small pieces..................oz.	8	12	16	20	24	36	8	8
Suspensory Bandages, cotton.............no.	4	8	12	16	20	36	4	8
Tape, cotton, or twilled stay binding...pieces.	3	6	9	12	15	30	3	3
woollen, or worsted binding.......pieces.	1	2	3	4	5	10	1	1
Thread, linen, unbleached.................oz.	2	3	4	5	6	12	2	1
Tow...lbs.	2	4	6	8	10	20	2	10
Towels.....................................doz.	5	10	15	20	25	50	5	2
Towels, roller.............................doz.	2	4	6	8	10	20	2	....
Twine, one half coarse.....................oz.	16	24	32	40	48	96	16	8
Books and Stationery, etc.								
Anatomy..............................copies.	1	1	1	1	1	1	1	....
Surgical, (of arteries,)............copies.	....	....	....	....	....	....	....	1
Chemistry............................copies.	1	1	1	1	1	1	1	....
Dictionary, Medical..................copies.	1	1	1	1	1	1	1	
Dictionary, English................copies.	1	1	1	1	1	1	1	....
Dispensatory.........................copies.	1	1	1	1	1	1	1	1
Hygiene..............................copies.	1	1	1	1	1	1	1	1
Jurisprudence........................copies.	1	1	1	1	1	1	1	....
Midwifery............................copies.	....	....	....	....	....	....	1	...

STANDARD SUPPLY TABLE.

ARTICLES.	ALLOWANCE FOR THREE MONTHS— For General Hospitals.						For a Reg't or 1,000 troops.	
	100 Beds.	200 Beds.	300 Beds.	400 Beds.	500 Beds.	1,000 Beds.	At Perm'nt Posts.	In the field
BOOKS AND STATIONERY, ETC.—Continued.								
Pathology ....copies.	1	1	1	1	1	1	1	....
Pharmacy ....copies.	1	1	1	1	1	1	1	....
Physiology ....copies.	1	1	1	1	1	1	1	....
Practice of Medicine ....copies.	2	2	2	2	2	2	2	....
Principles of Medicine ....copies.	1	1	1	1	1	1	1	....
Principles of Surgery ....copies.	1	1	1	1	1	1	1	....
Surgery—Macleod's Surgical Notes.copies.	1	1	1	1	1	1	1	....
Guthrie's Commentaries ....copies	1	1	1	1	1	1	1	....
Minor ....copies.	1	1	1	1	1	1	1	1
Therapeutics ....copies.	1	1	1	1	1	1	1	....
Longmore on Gunshot Wounds. ....copies.	1	1	1	1	1	1	1	...
Jones on Diseases of the Eye ....copies.	1	1	1	1	1	1	1	....
Toynbee on Diseases of the Ear ....copies.	1	1	1	1	1	1	1	....
Wilson on Diseases of the Skin ....copies.	1	1	1	1	1	1	1	....
Bumstead on Venereal Diseases ....copies.	1	1	1	1	1	1	1	....
Hospital Steward's Manual, Woodward's ....copies.	1	1	1	1	1	1	1	1
Blank Books, cap, half bound, 4 quires....no.	4	5	6	7	8	12	4	2
Case Book ....no.	1	1	1	1	2	2	1	....
Envelopes, printed, large 25, medium 25, small 50 ....no.	100	200	300	400	500	1000	100	100
Ink, 2 oz. bottles ....no.	3	6	9	12	15	24	6	2
Inkstands ....no.	2	2	3	3	4	4	2	....
Travelling ....no.	....	....	....	....	....	....	....	1
Meteorological Register ....no.	....	....	....	....	....	....	1	....
Morning Report Book, Regiment and Post.no.	1	1	1	1	1	1	1	1
General Hospital ....no.	1	1	1	1	1	1	1	1
Mucilage ....bottles.	1	1	2	2	3	4	1	1
Order and Letter Book ....no.	1	1	1	1	1	1	1	....
Prescription Book, Ward ....no.	2	4	6	8	10	20	2	2
Register of Patients ....no.	1	1	1	1	1	1	1	....
Regulations, Army ....copies.	1	1	1	1	1	1	1	....
Medical Department ....copies.	1	1	1	1	1	1	1	1
Paper, filtering, round, grey, 10 inches, .packs.	1	2	3	4	4	6	1	....
wrapping, white and blue ....quires.	4	6	8	10	12	24	4	2
writing, cap 1 quire, letter 1 quire, note 2 quires ....quires.	8	12	16	20	24	48	8	4
Pens, steel ....no.	24	36	48	60	72	144	24	24
Penholders ....no.	4	6	8	10	12	24	2	2
Pencils, lead, Faber's No. 2 ....no.	6	12	18	24	30	60	6	6
Portfolio, cap size ....no	1	1	1	1	1	1	1	1
Sealing Wax ....sticks.	1	2	3	4	5	10	1	1
BEDDING.								
Bed Sacks ....no.	112	224	336	448	560	1120	112	15
Beds, Water, of India-rubber ....no.	....	....	....	1	1	2	....	...
Blankets, white; grey for the field ....no.	200	400	600	800	1000	2000	200	20
Blanket cases, canvas ....no.		....	....	....	....	....	....	3
Counterpanes, according to pattern ....no.	112	224	336	448	560	1120	112	....

STANDARD SUPPLY TABLE.

Articles.	Allowance for three months— For General Hospitals.						For a Reg't or 1,000 troops.	
	100 Beds.	200 Beds.	300 Beds.	400 Beds.	500 Beds.	1,000 Beds.	At Perm'nt Posts.	In the field
Bedding.—Continued.								
Cushions, Rubber, for air, with open centre. no.	2	2	3	3	4	6	2	....
small..................... no.	4	4	6	6	8	12	4	....
Gutta-Percha Bed Covers, so made as to form, when united, a continuous covering.... no.	....	....	....	....	....	....	....	8
Mattresses, hair, in two equal parts, to pack folded..................... no.	10	20	30	40	50	100	10	....
of straw, moss, or shucks, in lieu of bed sacks, where they can be readily supplied..................... no.	100	200	300	400	500	1000	100	....
Musquito Bars, when specially required.... no.	100	200	300	400	500	1000	100	....
Pillows, hair..................... no.	112	224	336	448	560	1120	112	....
Pillow cases, cotton, colored.............. no.	....	....	...	...	....	....	....	15
linen, white..................... no.	148	296	444	592	740	1480	148	....
Ticks..................... no.	....	....	...	....	....	....	....	15
Sheets, linen..................... no.	400	800	1200	1600	2000	4000	400	....
Hospital Clothing.								
Caps, according to pattern.............. no.	100	200	300	400	500	1000	100	.. .
Drawers, according to pattern .... no.	200	400	600	800	1000	2000	200	....
Gowns, dressing, according to pattern..... no.	100	200	300	400	500	1000	100	....
Shirts, cotton, according to pattern ..... no.	200	400	600	800	1000	2000	200	....
Slippers, according to pattern............. no.	100	200	300	400	500	1000	100	....
Socks, woollen, according to pattern...... no.	200	400	600	800	1000	2000	200	....
Furniture and Appliances.								
Class No. 1.								
Basins, tin, small, for dressers........... no.	4	8	12	16	16	32	4	4
washhand..................... no.	10	20	30	40	50	100	10	4
Bed Pans, delf, shovel shape.............. no.	3	5	6	8	8	12	3	1
Screens..................... no.	2	4	6	8	10	20	2	...
Bedsteads, iron..................... no.	100	200	300	400	500	1000	100	....
Bedticket Frames..................... no.	100	200	300	400	500	100	100	....
Brooms..................... no.	4	8	12	16	20	40	4	....
Brushes, scrubbing..................... no.	4	8	12	16	20	40	4	....
Buckets, leather..................... no.	....	....	....	....	....	....	....	2
wooden..................... no.	4	8	12	16	20	40	4	....
Candlesticks..................... no.	4	16	24	30	36	72	8	....
Caldrons, with tin covers, 20 gallons....... no.	....	....	...	1	2	4	....	....
Chairs..................... no.	24	48	72	96	120	240	24	....
Clocks, wooden, small..................... no.	2	3	3	4	4	8	2	....
Clothes Line..................... feet.	300	500	700	900	1000	500	300	....
Closestools..................... no.	2	4	6	8	10	20	2	....
Corks, assorted..................... doz.	12	24	36	48	60	120	12	8
Corkscrews..................... no.	2	3	4	4	4	6	2	1
Feeding Cups, or sick feeders............. no.	4	6	8	10	12	18	4	...
Funnels. glass, ½ pint..................... no.	2	2	3	3	4	4	2	...
tin, pint..................... no.	2	2	3	3	4	4	2	1
Graters, nutmeg, and large.............. no.	2	2	2	3	3	6	2	1

STANDARD SUPPLY TABLE.

ARTICLES.	ALLOWANCE FOR THREE MONTHS—							
	For General Hospitals.						For a Reg't or 1,000 troops.	
	100 Beds.	200 Beds.	300 Beds.	400 Beds.	500 Beds.	1'000 Beds.	At Perm'nt Posts.	In the field
FURNITURE AND APPLIANCES—*Class No.* 1 Continued.								
Hatchet ....no.	1	1	2	2	3	3	1	1
Hone ....no.	1	1	1	1	1	1	1	1
Lanterns, glass ....no.	2	2	3	3	4	6	2	3
Litters, hand ....no.	4	4	4	4	6	6	4	4
horse ....no.	....	....	....	....	....	....	....	2
Looking-glasses, small ....no.	4	8	12	16	20	40	4	....
Measures, graduated, glass, 4 oz ....no.	2	3	4	4	5	6	2	1
minim ....no.	2	3	4	4	5	6	2	1
tin, gallon to pint ....no.	1	1	1	2	2	2	1	....
Medicine case, furnished by the list ....no.	....	....	....	....	....	....	....	2
Panniers, furnished by the list ....no.	....	....	....	....	....	....	....	2
Measuring Glasses ....no.	4	6	8	10	12	18	4	2
Spoons, delf ....no.	4	4	6	6	8	12	4	....
Mess Chest, furnished by list ....no.	....	....	....	....	....	....	....	1
Mortars and Pestles, wedgewood, 3½ to 8 inches ....no.	2	3	4	4	5	6	2	1
Pill Boxes, turned wood ....no.	4	6	8	10	12	18	4	2
Machine ....no.	1	1	1	2	2	2	1	....
Tiles, 5 to 10 inch ....no.	2	2	3	3	4	4	2	1
Pots, chamber, delf ....no.	10	20	30	40	50	100	10	....
inodorous, Army pattern ....no.	2	4	6	6	8	12	2	....
Rain Gauge ....no.	....	....	....	....	....	....	1	....
Range, size required, with fixtures complete ....no.	....	....	....	1	1	2	....	....
Razor and Strop, in case ....no.	1	1	2	2	3	4	1	1
Retort, delf, one quart ....no.	1	1	1	1	1	1	1	....
Sadirons ....no.	4	6	8	10	12	18	4	....
Scales and Weights, prescription ....no.	1	2	2	2	3	4	1	1
shop ....no.	1	1	1	1	1	2	1	....
Sheep Skins, dressed, for plasters ....no.	2	3	4	5	6	12	2	1
Slates ....no.	1	2	2	3	3	4	1	....
Spatulas, 3-inch and 6-inch ....no.	2	4	6	8	10	12	2	2
Spirit Lamp ....no.	1	1	1	1	2	2	1	....
Spit Mugs, without tops ....no.	6	10	14	18	24	36	6	....
Spittoons ....no.	12	24	36	48	60	120	12	....
Stoves, cooking size needed, with fixtures complete ....no.	1	1	2	....	....	....	1	....
Tables, bedside ....no.	50	100	150	200	250	500	50	....
Test Tubes ....no.	6	6	6	9	9	12	6	....
Thermometer and Hygrometer ....no.	1	1	1	1	1	1	1	....
Thermometer ....no.	1	1	1	2	2	2	1	....
Tin Warmer, for stomach, to hold hot water ....no.	1	1	1	1	2	2	1	....
for feet ....no.	1	1	2	2	3	4	1	....
Tubs, bath ....no.	1	1	2	2	3	4	1	....
Urinals, glass ....no.	2	4	6	8	10	18	2	2
Vials—6, 6-ounce; 12, 4-ounce; 3, 2-ounce; 3, 1-ounce ....doz.	8	16	24	32	40	72	8	2
Wood-saws ....no.	1	1	1	2	2	3	1	...

STANDARD SUPPLY TABLE.

ARTICLES.	ALLOWANCE FOR THREE MONTHS—							
	For General Hospitals.						For a Reg't or 1,000 troops.	
	100 Beds.	200 Beds.	300 Beds.	400 Beds.	500 Beds.	1,000 Beds.	At Perm'nt Posts.	In the field
FURNITURE AND APPLIANCES.—Continued.								
Class No. 2.								
Bowls, delf ... no.	60	120	180	240	300	600	60	....
Cleavers ... no.	1	1	1	2	2	3	1	....
Dippers, tin, pint size ... no.	2	4	6	8	10	18	2	....
Dishes, assorted sizes ... no.	14	20	26	32	38	48	14	....
Flesh Forks ... no.	1	1	1	2	2	3	1	....
Gridirons ... no.	2	2	2	3	3	4	2	....
Kettles, tea, iron ... no.	2	2	2	3	3	4	2	....
Knives and Forks, of each ... no.	60	120	180	240	300	600	60	....
carving, of each ... no.	2	4	6	6	8	12	2	....
Knives, bread ... no.	1	2	3	4	4	8	1	....
butchers ... no.	1	2	3	4	4	8	1	....
Ladles ... no.	2	2	2	3	3	4	2	....
Mugs, delf ... no.	60	120	180	240	300	600	60	....
Pans, frying ... no.	1	1	2	2	2	2	1	....
sauce ... no.	2	4	6	8	8	10	2	....
tin ... no.	2	2	3	3	4	6	2	....
Pitchers, delf, half gallon ... no.	6	12	18	24	30	60	6	....
Plates, delf ... no.	60	120	180	240	300	600	60	....
Pots, coffee, tin ... no.	4	6	8	10	12	24	4	....
mustard ... no.	2	4	6	8	10	20	2	....
pepper ... no.	2	4	6	8	10	20	2	....
tea, delf ... no.	4	6	8	10	12	24	4	....
Salt Cellars ... no.	6	12	18	24	30	60	6	....
Spoons, table ... no.	60	120	180	240	300	600	60	...
tea ... no.	60	120	180	240	300	600	60	....
Steel ... no.	1	1	2	2	3	4	1	....
Trays, butlers' ... no.	2	4	6	8	10	20	2	....
Tumblers, glass ... no.	12	24	36	48	60	120	12	....

ALLOWANCE OF SURGICAL INSTRUMENTS FOR MEDICAL OFFICERS.—FOR STAFF-SURGEONS AND ASSISTANT-SURGEONS.

For Capital Operations.

Two Amputating Knives, one long, one medium.
Two Catlings, one long, one medium.
Four Scalpels.
One Cartilage Knife.
One Capital Saw, long, bow, two blades.
One Metacarpal Saw.
One Chain Saw.
One Hey's Saw.
One Trephine, conical.
One Trephine, small crown.
One Bone Forceps, Liston's long, sharp, spring handle.
One Bone Forceps, broad-edged, slightly curved, spring handle.

One Bone Forceps, gnawing, spring handle.
One Bone Forceps, sequestrum, spring handle.
One Artery Forceps.
One Artery Needle.
One Artery Needle Key.
Twelve Surgeons' Needles.
One Tourniquet Screw, with pad.
One Tenaculum.
One Scissors.
One Chisel.
One Gouge.
One Mallet.
Four Drills (with one handle).
Two Retractors.
One Raspatory.
One Elevator.
One Brush.
Twelve yards Suture Wire, iron.
$\frac{1}{4}$ ounce Ligature Silk.
$\frac{1}{8}$ ounce Wax.
One Mahogany Case, brass bound, slide catch.
One Leather Pouch.

For Minor Operations.

One Amputating Knife.
Three Scalpels.
Two Bistouries.
One Hernia Knife.
One Finger Knife.
One Artery Forceps.
One Ball Forceps.
One Gullet Forceps.
One Dressing Forceps.
One Dissection Forceps.
One Artery Needle.
One Artery Needle Key.
Twelve Surgeons' Needles.
One Tenaculum.
Two Scissors.
One Trocar and Canula.
One Belloc's Canula.
One Bullet Probe.
One Director
One Cutting Pliers, small.
Six Steel Bougies, silvered, double curve, Nos. 1 and 2, 3 and 4, 5 and 6, 7 and 8, 9 and 10, 11 and 12.
Three Silver Catheters, Nos. 3, 6, and 9.
Six Gum-Elastic Catheters, Nos. 1, 3, 5, 7, 9, and 11.
Twenty-four Suture Pins, silvered.
Six yards Suture Wire, iron.
$\frac{1}{4}$ ounce Ligature Silk.
$\frac{1}{8}$ ounce Wax.
One Mahogany Case, brass-bound, slide catch.
One Leather Pouch.

For the Pocket Case.

One Scalpel.
Three Bistouries.
One Tenotome.
One Gum Lancet.
Two Thumb Lancets.
One Razor, small.
One Artery Forceps.
One Dressing Forceps.
One Artery Needle.
Six Surgeons' Needles.
One Exploring Needle.
One Tenaculum.
One Scissors.
One Director.
Three Probes.
One Caustic Holder.
One Silver Catheter, compound.
Six yards Suture Wire, iron.
$\frac{1}{4}$ ounce Ligature Silk.
$\frac{1}{8}$ ounce Wax.
One Russia Leather Case.

One Leather Trunk for the set.

FOR REGIMENTAL-SURGEONS AND ASSISTANT-SURGEONS.

For the Field Case.

Two Amputating Knives, one long, one medium.
Two Catlings, one long, one medium.
Three Scalpels.
Two Bistouries.
One Hernia Knife.
One Finger Knife.
One Capital Saw, long, bow, two blades.
One Metacarpal Saw.
One Hey's Saw.
One Trephine, conical.
One Bone Forceps, broad-edged, slightly curved, spring handle.
One Bone Forceps, sequestrum, spring handle.
One Artery Forceps.
One Ball Forceps.
One Dressing Forceps.
One Dissection Forceps.
One Artery Needle.
One Artery Needle Key.
Twelve Surgeons' Needles.
One Tourniquet, screw, with pad.
One Tenaculum.
Two Scissors.
Two Retractors.
One Trocar and Canula.
One Raspatory.
One Elevator.
One Brush.
One Bullet Probe.
One Director.
Six Steel Bougies, silvered, double curve, Nos, 1 and 2, 3 and 4, 5 and 6, 7 and 8, 9 and 10, 11, and 12.
Three Silver Catheters, Nos. 3, 6, 9.
Six Gum-Elastic Catheters, Nos. 1, 3, 5, 7, 9, 11.
Twelve yards Suture Wire, iron.
¼ ounce Ligature Silk.
½ ounce Wax.
One Mahogany Case, brass-bound, slide catch.
One Leather Pouch.

Pocket Case the same as allowed to Staff-Surgeons.

CONTENTS OF THE SETS OF INSTRUMENTS AND APPLIANCES REFERRED TO IN THE STANDARD SUPPLY TABLE.

1. *The Dissecting Case.*

One Cartilage Knife.
Three Scalpels.
One Tenaculum.
One Dissection Forceps.
One Chain and Hooks.
Two Needles and Thread.
One Enterotome.
One Scissors.
One Blowpipe.
One Chisel.
Mahogany Box.

2. *The Obstetrical Case.*

One Simpson's Forceps.
One Vectis or Lever.
One Crochet and Blunt Hook.
One Perforator.
Russia Leather Case.

3. *The Pocket Case for Hospitals.*

One sharp-pointed Bistoury.
One probe-pointed Bistoury.
One Scalpel.
One Tenaculum.

One Abscess Lancet.
One Compound Catheter.
One Straight Scissors.
One Angular Scissors.
One Dressing Forceps.
One Artery Forceps.
One Spatula.
One Director.
Two Probes.
Six Needles.
Ligature Silk and Wax.
Russia Leather Case.

4. *The Teeth-Extracting Case.*

One Key with three Hooks.
Two Forceps for Molars.
One Forceps for Bicuspids.
One Forceps for Incisors.
One Gum Lancet.
One Stump Elevator.
Russia Leather Case.

5. *The Medicine Case for Field Service.*

Chloroformum Purificatum,	oz.	6½
Extractum Ipecacuanhæ Fluidum,	oz.	2
Extract. Zingiberis Fluidum,	oz.	2
Liquor Ferri Persulphatus,	oz.	2
Pilulæ Catharticæ Compositæ,	doz.	12
Pilulæ Quiniæ Sulphatis (3 grains each),	doz.	12
Pilulæ Opii,	doz.	12
Pills of Ext. Colocyn. Comp. 3 grs., and Ipecac. ½ gr.,	doz.	12
Spiritus Frumenti,	f℥	24
Tinctura Opii,	"	2
Corks,	no.	6
Ichthyocolla Plaster,	yard	1
Lint, patent, "A. super,"	lb.	¼
Medicine Glass,	no.	1
Muslin, Bleached, one yard wide,	yards	2
Pins,	paper	1
Roller Bandages,	no.	24
Scissors,	pair	1
Silk for Ligatures,	oz.	¼
Sponge, fine, small,	piece	1
Spoon, tea, tinned iron,	no.	1
Towel,	no.	1

6. *The Medicine Pannier.*

Each Pannier contains as follows:

Medicines, &c.

Acidum Tannicum,	oz.	½
Alcohol Fortius,	f℥	12
Alumen,	oz.	3
Antimonii et Potassæ Tartras,	oz.	1
Argenti Nitras,	oz.	1
Argenti Nitras Fusus,	oz.	1
Capsici Pulvis,	oz.	1
Ceratum Adipis,	oz.	16
Ceratum Cantharidis,	oz.	3
Chloroformum Purificatum,	f℥	12
Collodium,	"	3
Cough Mixture,	"	12
Creasotum,	f℥	2
Extractum Aconiti Radicis Fluidum,	"	3
Extract. Cinchonæ Fluidum (with Aromatics),	"	4
Extractum Colchici Seminis Fluidum,	"	3
Extractum Ipecacuanhæ Fluidum,	"	3
Extract. Valerianæ Fluidum,	"	6
Extract. Zingiberis Fluidum,	"	6
Glycerina,	"	6
Iodinium,	oz.	1

Liniment,	f℥	12
Liquor Ammoniæ,	"	8
Liquor Ferri Persulphatis,	"	4
Morphiæ Sulphas (in solution 16 grs. to the f℥),	"	4
Oleum Olivæ,	"	6
Oleum Terebinthinæ,	"	6
Pilulæ Catharticæ Compositæ,	doz.	50
Pilulæ Hydrargyri,	doz.	40
Pilulæ Opii,	doz.	60
Pilulæ Quiniæ Sulphatis (3 grs. each),	doz.	40
Pills of Camphor 2 grs., and Opium 1 gr.,	doz.	20
Pills of Ext. Colocyn. Comp. 3 grs., Ipecac. ½ gr.	doz.	50
Pills of Pulv. Ipecac. et Opii (5 grs. each),	doz.	30
Plumbi Acetas,	oz.	3
Potassæ Bicarbonas,	oz.	4
Potassæ Chloras,	oz.	4
Potassii Iodidum,	oz.	4
Sapo,	cake	1
Sodæ et Potassæ Tartras,	oz.	4
Spiritus Ammoniæ Aromaticus,	f℥	4
Spiritus Ætheris Compositus,	"	4
Spiritus Ætheris Nitrici,	"	8
Spiritus Frumenti,	"	24
Syrupus Scillæ,	"	8
Tinctura Ferri Chloridi,	"	2
Tinctura Opii,	"	6
Tinctura Opii Camphorata,	"	6
Unguentum Hydrargyri,	oz.	6
Zinci Sulphas,	oz.	3

Hospital Stores.

Beef, extract of,	lb.	1
Candles, composition, half-length,	lb.	½
Coffee, extract of,	lb.	1
Milk, condensed,	lb.	1
Sugar, white, kiln-dried,	oz.	10
Tea, black,	oz.	4

Instruments.

Cupping Tins,	no.	4
Probang,	no.	1
Scissors,	pair	1
Syringes, self-injecting,	no.	1
Syringes, penis, glass, in cases,	no.	4
Tourniquets, field,	no.	2

Dressings, &c.

Adhesive Plaster, in tin cans,	yards	2
Binders' Boards,	pieces	8
Icthyocolla Plaster,	yard	1
Lint, patent, "A. super,"	lb.	½
Matches,	box.	1
Muslin, Bleached, 1 yard wide,	yards	3
Needles, 25; Cotton, 1 spool; Thimble, 1, in case,	no.	1
Oiled Silk,	yard	⅞
Pencils, hair, in vial,	no.	6
Pins,	paper	1
Roller Bandages:		
6—1 in. by 1 yd. long,		3 doz.
12—2 ins. by 3 yds. long,		
12—2½ ins. by 3 yds. long,		
4—3 ins. by 4 yds. long,		
1—3½ ins. by 5 yds. long,		
1—4 ins. by 8 yds. long,		
Silk, Saddlers', for ligatures,	oz.	¼
Sponge, fine, small pieces,	no.	6
Tape, pieces,	pieces	2
Tow,	lb.	1
Towels,	no.	3

Books, &c.

Morning Report Book,	no.	1
Register and Prescription Book,	no.	1
Envelopes, printed, letter size,	no.	25

Inkstand, travellers', filled,	no.	1
Paper, note, ruled,	quires	2
Pens, Gillott's steel, gilt, in box,	no.	12
Penholders,	no.	3
Pencils, lead, Faber's, No. 2,	no.	2
Tray, tin, for books and stationery,	no.	1

Furniture, &c.

Basins, small tin, for dressing,	no.	2
Candle-Holder,	no.	1
Corks,	doz.	4
Corkscrew,	no.	1
Measure, graduated glass, 2 f℥,	no.	1
Measure, graduated glass, minim,	no.	1
Medicine Measuring Glass, in case,	no.	1
Mortar and Pestle,	no.	1
Pill Boxes,	paper	4½
Scales and Weights, prescription,	set	1
Spatula, riveted handle, 3-inch,	no.	1
Spoon, tea, tinned iron,	no.	1
Vials: 2—4-ounce, 2—2-ounce, 2—1-ounce,	no.	6

7. *The Hospital Mess-Chest.*

Six Tin Basins, small.
Two Tin Basins, Washstand.
Two Boxes for Pepper and Salt.
Six Tin Cups.
Four Canisters, for Tea, Coffee, Sugar, and Butter.
Two Dippers and Ladles.
One Grater.
One Iron Pot.
One Tin Coffee Pot.
One Tin Tea Pot.
Six Tin Tumblers.
One Iron Tea-kettle.
One Gridiron.
Twelve Knives and Forks.
Six half-pint Britannia Mugs.
One Frying-Pan.
One Sauce Pan.
Six Tin Plates.
Two Tin Dishes.
Six Iron Table Spoons, tinned.
Six Iron Teaspoons, tinned.
One Tin Tray.

WILLIAM A. HAMMOND,
Surgeon-General U. S. Army.

NOTES.

1. The materials for preparing CHLORINIUM are a Sulphuric Acid Mixture and a Common Salt Mixture.

The Sulphuric Acid Mixture.

Take of Sulphuric Acid S.G. 1845........................45 parts.
Water..21 parts.

Mix them carefully, and when cold put the mixture into strong bottles with accurately ground stoppers, each bottle to contain sixty-five fluid ounces.

Half a fluid ounce of this to be used for each package of the Common Salt Mixture.

The Common Salt Mixture.

Take of Common Salt, well dried.......................1800 parts.
Binoxide of Manganese, containing 72 per cent.......1875 parts.

Grind them together into a fine powder, and put the powder up in packages containing about 195 grains each, and put 130 of these packages in a pasteboard box, to accompany the Sulphuric Acid Mixture.

Each of these packages requires half a fluid ounce of the Sulphuric Acid Mixture, and yields about 57 cubic inches of Chlorine. This quantity, when thus liberated gradually in a space containing about 20,000 times its volume of air, is borne without inconvenience by persons generally, and is not injurious even in pulmonary diseases. As very much depends upon the ventilation of apartments wherein it is to be used, no absolute rules of application can be laid down, except that it should never be used in such quantities as to produce discomfort or bronchial irritation to patients.

DIRECTIONS FOR USE.

One of the above packages or papers of the Common Salt Mixture placed in a saucer or plate, and thoroughly mixed with half a fluid ounce of the Sulphuric Acid Mixture, is to be placed under every alternate bed at night, and allowed to remain there three days Upon the second night the beds which were omitted the first night should be supplied in the same way, and for the same length of time; and the whole process repeated at the end of three days, or sooner, according to circumstances. Should the wards be badly ventilated or contain many sloughing wounds, or be subject to epidemic disease or low forms of fever, the process should be continuous—that is, the mixture should be renewed every third day. Otherwise, once or twice a month may be sufficient. And when thorough cleanliness and ventilation are attained, the process is unnecessary for occupied wards.

In disinfecting unoccupied wards, water closets, latrines, etc., by Chlorine, they should be first cleansed, be closed up as perfectly as practicable, and two packages used for each 600 cubic feet of space.

2. The "Cough Mixture" consists of Syrup of Squills and Camphorated Tincture of Opium, each four fluid ounces, with two fluid drachms of Fluid Extract of Ipecacuanha. The dose is one teaspoonful.

3. The "Liniment" is prepared with equal parts of Water of Ammonia, Oil of Turpentine, and Olive Oil.

FORM 1.

Summary statement of funds received, disbursed, and transferred at ——, *by* [here insert name, rank, and title,] *United States Army, during the month of* ——, 186 .

DR. CR.

186 .		Dolls.	Cts.	186 .		Dolls.	Cts.
	To amount disbursed this month...........				By balance, per last Summary Statement...		
	To transfer to ——......................				By cash from ——		
	To balance due United States...............						
	$				$		

I certify on honor that the above is a true statement of all moneys on hand at last statement, received, disbursed, or transferred during the month on account of the Medical Department of the Army, and that the balance of —— dollars and —— cents is deposited with the United States Treasurer at ——, with the exception of —— dollars and —— cents, in my hands in United States Treasury notes and in ——.

—— ——,
—— ——,
United States Army.

NOTE.—*Vouchers* for money disbursed or transferred *do not* accompany the Summary Statement. Triplicates—one for the Second Auditor, one for the Surgeon-General, and one to be retained.

Indorsement to be as follows :

Summary Statement of Funds.
Station.
Period.
Date.

—— ——,
United States Army

Form 2.

Estimate of funds required for the service of the Medical Department at ——, *by* [here insert name, rank, and title,] *United States Army, in the month ending* —— —, 186 .

		Dollars.	Cents.
1	For medicines, instruments, dressing, &c.		
2	For hospital stores, bedding, &c.		
3	For hospital furniture and field equipments.		
4	For medical books, stationery, and printing.		
5	For private physicians and medicine furnished by them.		
6	For hire of clerks and laborers in purveying depôts.		
7	For pay to soldiers acting as cooks and nurses.		
8	For ice, fruits, and other comforts.		
9	For citizen nurses.		
10	For hospital clothing.		
11	For care of sick soldiers in private hospitals.		
12	For artificial limbs.		
13	For outstanding debts.		
	Deduct actual or probable balance on hand.		
	Amount required. $		

—— ——,
United States Army.

Indorsement to be as follows:

Estimate of Funds.
Station.
Period.
Date.

—— ——,
United States Army.

Form 3.

The United States in account current with [here insert the name, rank, and title,] *United States Army, for expenditures on account of the Medical Department in the quarter ending* ——— —, 186 .

Dr. Cr.

186 .		Dollars.	Cents.	186 .		Dollars.	Cents.
	To amount of expenditures, per abstract of disbursements........................				By balance on hand per last account......		
	To balance due the United States, carried to new account				By cash received from Treasurer of the United States, being amount of Warrant No.		
					By cash received from sales of public property as per account herewith..........		
	$				$		

I certify on honor that the above account current exhibits an accurate and true statement of all moneys received and expended by me on account of the Medical Department of the army not heretofore accounted for, and that the balance of ——— dollars and ——— cents due the United States by me is deposited with the United States Assistant Treasurer at ———, except the sum of ——— dollars and ——— cents in my hands in United States Treasury notes and in ———

——— ———,
Medical Purveyor United States Army.

Notes.—*Vouchers* for money disbursed and transferred during the quarter must accompany this *Quarterly Account Current.*
Money accounts should be kept open *till the end of the quarter*, unless an officer ceases to do duty in the department.

Indorsement to be as follows:

Quarterly Account Current.
Station ———,
Period ———,
Date ———,

——— ———,
——— ——— *U. S. Army.*

FORM 4.

Abstract of disbursements on account of the Medical Department by [here insert name, rank, and title,] *United States Army, at* ———, *in the quarter ending* ———, 186 .

Date of payment.	No. of Voucher.	To whom paid.	On what account.	Dollars.	Cents.
			$		

I certify on honor that the above abstract is correct.

—— ——,
United States Army.

Indorsement to be as follows :

Abstract of disbursements.
Station ———.
Period ———.
Date ———.

—— ——,
United States Army.

$ —— ——.

FORM 5.

The United States to ——— ———, Dr.

Date.	Articles.	Quantity.	Price.	Dollars.	Cents.
1863. Jan. 26.	Chloroformum .... oz.	12	$0 18	2	16
	Pilulæ Quiniæ Sulphatis (3 grs. each)........ doz.	40	0 36	14	40
	Quiniæ Sulphatis........ oz.	100	2 30	230	00
				246	56

Received [here insert place and date], 186 , of [here insert name, rank, and title,] U. S. Army, two hundred and forty-six dollars and fifty-six cents, in full of the above account.

Signed duplicates.

——— ———.

Indorsements to be as follows :
Voucher No. —.
Name ——— ———.
Articles of service ———.
Date ———.
$ ———.

FORM 6.

Return of medical and hospital property received, expended, issued, and remaining on hand at ——— ———, for the ——— ending ———, 186- .

Articles and quantities.		On hand at last return.	Received since last return.	Total to be accounted for.	Expended with the sick.	Issued.	Lost or destroyed by unavoidable accident.	Worn out, or unfit for use.	Total expended, issued, &c.	On hand.	Remarks.
Materia Medica.											
Acaciæ Pulvis,	oz.	32	56	88	56	16	0	0	72	16	
Acidum Aceticum,	oz.	8	16	24	8	0	0	0	8	16	
Acidum Citricum,	oz.	16	48	64	16	0	0	16	32	32	Condemned and ordered to be dropped. See inclosed report.
Acidum Muriaticum,	oz.	40	40	80	16	16	24	0	56	24	Bottle broken; acid lost.

I certify on honor that the above return is correct, to the best of my knowledge, and that the medicines and stores have been expended with the sick belonging to the army alone.

——— ———,
Surgeon United States Army.

N.B.—Returns will always be transmitted in duplicate, and by different mails. Articles purchased with the *Hospital Fund* will not be accounted for on this return. No officer shall drop from his return any public property as worn out or unserviceable until it has been condemned after proper inspection and ordered to be so dropped.

FORM 7.

Abstract of medical and hospital property received and issued at ————, *in the* ————, *ending on the* —— *day of* ———, 186 , *by* [here insert name, rank, and title,] *U. S. Army.*

Articles and quantities.	RECEIVED FROM.						ISSUED TO.								
	Voucher No. 1. (Name.)	Voucher No. 2. (Name.)	Voucher No. 3. (Name.)	Voucher No. 4. (Name.)	Voucher No. 5. (Name.)	Total.	Voucher No. 1. (Name.)	Voucher No. 2. (Name.)	Voucher No. 3. (Name.)	Voucher No. 4. (Name.)	Voucher No. 5. (Name.)	Voucher No. 6. (Name.)	Voucher No. 7. (Name.)	Voucher No. 8. (Name.)	Total.
Materia Medica.															
Acaciæ Pulvis..................oz.															
Acidum Aceticum...............oz.															

I certify that the above abstract is correct.

—— ——,

————, *U. S. Army.*

N.B.—Invoices and receipts must accompany this abstract. When the receipts and issues are numerous, a separate abstract may be made for each.

FORM 8.

Requisition for medical and hospital supplies.

Station, ——— ——— ———. Period, ——— ——— ———.
From ——— ——— ——— to ——— ——— ———.
Command: Officers, ———; Enlisted Men, ———; All others entitled to Medicines, ———; Total, ———.

Articles and quantities.	On hand.	Wanted.	Articles and quantities.	On hand.	Wanted.
Materia Medica.					
Acaciæ Pulvis..................oz.					
Acidum Aceticum..................oz.					

Date, ——— ———.

——— ———,
Surgeon U. S. Army.

N.B.—Requisitions will exhibit the quantity of each article "on hand" of which more is "wanted." They will be transmitted in duplicate, and by different mails.

Indorsement to be as follows:

Requisition.
Station, ——— ———.
Period, ——— ———.
From ——— ———.
To ——— ———.
——— ———,
———, *U. S. Army.*

——— ———,
———, *U. S. Army.*

Form 9.

Special requisition on the Quartermaster's Department for medical and hospital supplies required at ——.

Ammoniæ Carbonas..oz. 32
Quiniæ Sulphas..oz. 10
&c. &c.
&c. &c.

I certify that the medicines above required are necessary for the sick at ——, in consequence of, [here state whether from loss, damage, &c., &c.,] and that the requisition is agreeable to the Supply Table, and that recourse cannot be had to a Medical Purveyor or Storekeeper in time to meet the emergency.

—— ——,
Surgeon United States Army.

Approved:

—— ——,
Commanding Officer.

Received —— —, 186 , of ——, the articles above enumerated.

—— ——,
Surgeon United States Army.

Form 10.

Account for medicines, &c., purchased by an officer of the Quartermaster's Department.

The United States *To* —— —— Dr.

	Quantity.	Price.	Dolls.	Cts.
Ammoniæ Carbonas....................oz.	32	$0 04	1	28
Quiniæ Sulphas........................oz.	10	2 95	29	50
			30	78

I certify that the articles above charged for the use of the sick at —— are agreeable to the foregoing requisition, and that the charges are reasonable and just.

—— ——,
Surgeon United States Army.

Received, —— ——, 186 , of ——, —— dollars and — cents, in full of the above account.

—— ——.

Note.—The above certificate may be signed by the Surgeon making the requisition, or by any Surgeon or Assistant-Surgeon belonging to the army.

Signed triplicates.

Form 11.

Annual return of surgical instruments in the possession of ——— ——— *Medical Department, United States Army, on the* — *day of December,* 186 .

For capital operations.	No.	Condition.	For minor operations.	No.	Condition.	For the pocket case.	No.	Condition.	For the field case.	No.	Condition.

I certify on honor that this return is correct, and that the surgical instruments were issued to me by ——— ——— on the — day of ———, 186 , for my personal use, agreeably to the regulations for the Medical Department of the army.

——— ———,
Surgeon United States Army.

Note.—The true condition of each instrument must be stated, and if any be lost or damaged a report of the facts and circumstances attending such loss or damage must be given. A duplicate of this return is required.

CIRCULAR No. 8.

Surgeon-General's Office,
Washington, *June* 22, 1863.

I. It is provided, by Act of Congress, that soldiers discharged from the Army of the United States *within two years* from the date of their enlistment *by reason of wounds received in battle*, shall be entitled to receive the same bounty as is granted to those discharged *after two* years' service.

Medical Officers are accordingly directed, in making out the papers of soldiers discharged under such circumstances, to endorse upon both the Final Statements and the Discharge the fact that the disability is by reason of wounds received in battle, and to sign such endorsement with their official signature.

II. Hereafter in giving Discharges to officers and soldiers on account of disability, their discharge papers must always state whether, at the time of discharge, the officer or soldier was or was not physically suitable to enter or re-enlist in the Invalid Corps.

III. From and after the 30th instant, the envelopes of all official communications addressed to the heads of bureaux of the War Department having the franking privilege, must be marked "Official," with the signature thereto of the officer writing the communication. Postage stamps are not required on such communications.

WILLIAM A. HAMMOND,
Surgeon-General.

CIRCULAR No. 10.

Surgeon-General's Office,
Washington, *July* 15, 1863.

Surgeons in charge of U. S. Hospitals will forward to this Office, without delay, rolls of all Prisoners of War now inmates of their hospitals, or who may be hereafter received as such.

These rolls will contain the names, rank, company, and regiment of the prisoners, and the time and place of their capture.

WILLIAM A. HAMMOND,
Surgeon-General.

CIRCULAR No. 11.

Surgeon-General's Office,
Washington, *July* 25, 1863.

In the examination of soldiers for the "Invalid Corps," Surgeons in charge of Hospitals and Convalescent Camps will be guided by the following instructions, in addition to orders already issued by the War Department:

Whenever a Board is ordered to a Hospital or Convalescent Camp for the purpose of examining men for the Invalid Corps, all Medical Officers thereat will furnish every facility to the Board in the prosecution of its duties—giving, in every case, such information as may be in their power to give concerning the Military History and Records of those under their charge.

Clerical aid will be furnished to the Boards, upon their request, from soldiers in Hospital, by the Surgeon in charge.

These Boards being governed in their duties by General Orders from the War Department, and special instructions from the Provost-Marshal-General, no obstruction will be offered to the prompt performance of their duty; and Medical Officers will in no case interfere with or attempt to assume control over the Board, or any individual member thereof.

WILLIAM A. HAMMOND,
Surgeon-General.

CIRCULAR No. 12.

Surgeon-General's Office,
Washington, *July* 29, 1863.

The attention of Medical Officers is called to the virtues of Permanganate of Potassa as a disinfectant and deodorizer.

A preparation of this salt in solution is supplied by the Medical Department. Medical Officers are directed to make proper requisitions therefor upon Medical Purveyors whenever its use may be indicated; and Medical Purveyors and Storekeepers are directed to keep a stock on hand by making timely requisition on this Office.

WILLIAM A. HAMMOND,
Surgeon-General.

CIRCULAR No. 13.

Surgeon-General's Office,
Washington, *August* 15, 1863.

Surgeons in charge of Hospitals are informed that they may procure a substitute for *Port Wine*, for the use of the sick, by making proper requisition therefor.

In consequence of the impossibility of procuring pure Port Wine of the grade formerly issued to the Army, an article of Tarragona wine has been adopted for issue instead.

This wine is light, dry, and adstringent, and is the pure juice of the grape, purchased by the Medical Department in bond, and bottled at Medical Purveying establishments.

WILLIAM A. HAMMOND,
Surgeon-General.

CIRCULAR No. 14.

Surgeon-General's Office,
Washington, *August* 16, 1863.

Upon the Monthly Statement of the Hospital Fund required to be forwarded to this Office, Surgeons in charge of Hospitals will hereafter endorse the name, rank, and station of the Commissary of Subsistence by whom the Hospital rations are issued.

As large Hospital Funds have accrued and remained unexpended in a few instances, Surgeons in charge of Hospitals whose funds may be from any cause insufficient, are directed to apply to this office for the transfer of a sufficient sum to meet their necessities. The application must state the amount needed, and the specified purpose for which needed, and the circumstances causing the necessity. If the reasons given are satisfactory, the transfer asked will be made

WILLIAM A. HAMMOND,
Surgeon-General.

CIRCULAR No. 16.

Surgeon-General's Office,
Washington, D. C., *Sept.* 12, 1863.

The attention of all Medical Directors is especially called to Paragraph 169, Revised U. S. Regulations, and Section II., General Orders, No. 98, dated Head-Quarters of the Army, Adjutant-General's Office, November 13, 1861, in regard to the disposition to be made of "Insane Soldiers."

No insane soldier can be discharged the service on Surgeon's Certificate of Disability.

JOSEPH K. BARNES,
Acting Surgeon-General.

CIRCULAR NO. 17.

Surgeon-General's Office,
Washington, D.C., *September* 14, 1863.

Medical Directors are hereby instructed that, in obedience to an order from the War Department, *all* enlisted men of the Regular Regiments (excepting Hospital Stewards) now employed in Hospitals, must be at once sent to their respective regiments.

By order:

CHAS. S. CRANE,
Surgeon, U. S. Army.

CIRCULAR NO. 18.

Surgeon-General's Office,
Washington, D.C., *September* 16, 1863.

The following construction of the new postal law relative to the weight of packages which may be sent by mail, free of postage, is published for the information of the officers of the Medical Department, especially Medical Directors and Purveyors:

"Post Office Department,
"Appointment Office, *September* 8, 1863.

* * * * * * * * * * *

"The maximum weight of packages which may be sent through the mails is limited to 'four' pounds, except Congressional documents and books published or purchased by order of Congress. It was not the intention of the law to prescribe a smaller limit to franked packages to or from any of the Executive Departments and Bureaus, as that would exclude from the mails a large portion of the official correspondence of the Government.

* * * * * * * * * * *

(Signed)

"ALEX. W. RANDALL,
"*First Assistant Postmaster-General.*"

By order:

C. H. CRANE,
Surgeon, U. S. Army.

CIRCULAR NO. 19.

Surgeon-General's Office,
Washington, D.C., *September* 25, 1863.

Hereafter, in the "Monthly Statement of Hospital Fund" forwarded to this office, an entry must be made of the outstanding and *unpaid* debts that are chargeable against such fund. Only the sum total of the indebtedness, and not the items in detail, is required.

Attention is called to Circular No. 14, from this office, date of August 16, 1863, requiring the name, rank, etc., of the Commissary of Subsistence, by whom the Hospital rations are issued, to be endorsed on each Monthly Statement of Hospital Fund.

A well-organized General Hospital, under ordinary circumstances, should never be in debt, as it is believed that the *fund* monthly accruing from the savings on rations will be ample to cover all the legitimate expenditures for articles authorized to be purchased with such *fund;* and the Surgeons in charge will hereafter be held to a strict accountability for the proper and economical management of their "Hospital Fund."

By order:

C. H. CRANE,
Surgeon, U. S. Army.

CIRCULAR NO. 19½.

Surgeon-General's Office,
Washington, D.C., *September* 28, 1863.

The assignment of officers in command of companies of the Invalid Corps to General Hospitals, is for the purpose of increasing the efficiency of the Hospitals, and is a part of the Hospital organization, under the Senior Medical Director.

They are, while on that duty, a portion of the Commissioned Staff of the Hospital, and are entitled to the same allowance of quarters, fuel, etc., within the Hospital, when at all practicable, as Medical Officers of similar rank.

It is confidently expected that much benefit will be derived from the provisions of General Orders No. 212, current series, and that Surgeons in charge of General Hospitals will endeavor to render the position of these officers such that there will be entire harmony and concord of action in the performance of their respective duties.

By order:

C. H. CRANE,
Surgeon, U. S. A.

CIRCULAR NO. 20.

Surgeon-General's Office,
Washington City, D.C., *Sept.* 29, 1863.

Medical Directors, in cities where there are several General Hospitals, will designate one in each city, at which enlisted men requiring trusses. will report themselves to the Surgeon in charge, to be measured for and fitted with the proper instruments. Medical Purveyors will cause to be made, and furnish, trusses corresponding in measure and description with the requisition to be made in each case, in lieu of the usual issue, which will be discontinued to all General Hospitals where this arrangement can be carried into effect.

By order:

C. H. CRANE,
Surgeon, U. S. Army.

CIRCULAR No. 21.

Surgeon-General's Office,
Washington, D.C., *October* 1, 1863.

The following instructions, concerning the manner of making out the "Accounts of Private Physicians under Contract," are issued for the benefit of all concerned:

1st. Accounts must be made out for periods of one or more complete months, commencing with the date of entry upon service. No account embracing fractional periods of a month will receive attention, unless it appears upon the face of the account either that the station of the physician has been changed or his contract annulled.

2d. Officers certifying to accounts of a "private physician under contract," must give their official title, and state explicitly the capacity in which they are serving; otherwise their authority to make such a certificate may be questioned. E. g., A. B., Surgeon U. S. A., *in charge* ——— *General Hospital.* C. D., Surg. Vols., *Medical Director*, 1*st Division*, 2*d Army Corps.* E. F., Col. 40th Ohio Vols.; *Commanding Post, Garrison, or Regiment.*

3d. The Hospital, Post, Regiment, or Camp in which the services are rendered, must be explicitly stated, and the strength of the command also noted.

4th. When accounts are certified to by a Line Officer commanding a Post, Regiment, or Camp, they must be transmitted to this Office, through the Department Medical Director, and receive his approval.

5th. The mere approval of an account will not secure its passage through the Treasury. The signature of the certifying officer must be placed in the blank space *immediately below the certificate*, and not, as now frequently occurs, in some other part of the account, thus leaving the certificate unsigned.

6th. The dates between which the services are rendered must be accurately stated. Both the *initial and final day* are counted; thus, from "August 20, 1863, to September 20, 1863, inclusive," is not one month, but one month and one day. It should read, "from August 20, 1863, to September 19, 1863, inclusive," being *one* month.

7th. When instruments are furnished to a Contract Physician by a Medical Purveyor, the kind, and cost price thereof, are to be reported by the Medical Purveyor to this office. The cost price is then deducted from the first account for services rendered subsequent to such reports. The instruments then become the private property of the Contract Physician, and are in no case to be turned back to a Purveyor or other officer without the written order of this office.

8th. When a Contract Physician has been absent from duty, the certifying officer must state the reason and duration thereof.

Contract Physicians are requested to use the blank printed accounts furnished by this office; an abundant supply of which will be issued to every hospital, post, etc., on the request of the Surgeon in Charge or Commanding Officer.

Contract Physicians, who desire it, can have their certificates made payable to any person besides themselves, by simply endorsing on the face of the account:

"Pay to the order of ——— ———

(Signature.) ——— ———,
"*Acting Ass't Surgeon, U. S. A.*"

The certificate will then be made out in accordance with such order, and the payee has only to prove his identity in order to receive the money.

The numerous and embarrassing delays in this class of accounts abundantly prove that too great care cannot be exercised, both by the certifying officer and the physician in whose name the account is rendered.

JOSEPH K. BARNES,
Acting Surgeon-General.

CIRCULAR No. 22.

Surgeon-General's Office.
Washington, D.C., *October* 10, 1863.

The following letter from the Provost-Marshal-General is published for the information of the Medical Officers of the Army:

"War Department, Provost-Marshal-General's Office,
Washington, D.C., *October* 9, 1863.

"COLONEL: I have the honor to return the inclosed communication from Medical-Inspector Cuyler, and beg leave to state that the Surgeons in charge of Hospitals are directed in Paragraph VI. General Order, No. 212, to forward to this Bureau rolls of all men reported by them for transfer to Invalid Corps, after each regular muster. Immediately on the receipt of these rolls in this Bureau, the Acting Assistant Provost-Marshal-General of the State in which the Hospital is located, is notified to receive the men whose names are on the rolls, and assign them to Companies in the Battalion to which they are reported to belong by the Surgeon. Should any of the men recommended by him (the Surgeon) for the 2d Battalion be needed in the Hospital for nurses, cooks, etc., they will be at once assigned to such duty. Full companies can be organized in Hospitals where their services are needed, and officers will be assigned to command them, and will clothe, arm, and equip the men.

"Where no Companies exist in a State from which rolls are received from a Surgeon, then the Provost-Marshal of the State is ordered to receive the men and hold them as a nucleus for the formation of a Company.

"The names of the men thus reported are published in a General Order, which completes their transfer to the Corps. The necessity for subsisting the men must necessarily exist until an officer is assigned to command them, when provisions will be drawn on a regular Company Return by that officer.

"As the number of officers of the Corps is limited, and by no means adequate to its requirements at present, it is confidently expected that the Surgeons will accord to us that patience and forbearance which we are led to expect from the great courtesy and hearty coöperation with which they have already favored the corps.

"I am, very respectfully,
"Your obedient servant,
"JAMES B. FRY,
"*Provost-Marshal-General.*

"Colonel BARNES,
"*Acting Surgeon-General,*
"*United States Army.*"

By order of the Acting Surgeon-General:

C. H. CRANE,
Surgeon, U. S. A.

CIRCULAR No. 23.

Surgeon-General's Office,
Washington, D.C., *October* 17, 1863.

" Office of Commissary-General of Prisoners,
" Washington, D.C., *October* 17, 1863.

"COLONEL: I have the honor to request that orders may be given to the Surgeons in charge of the various Hospitals at which Prisoners of War are held, to furnish this office with a semi-monthly report of deceased prisoners—reports to be furnished on the fifteenth and last days of each month—giving rank, regiment, company, date and place of capture, date of decease, cause, place of interment, number of grave, and, if practicable, any information necessary to trace their place of burial.

"It is desired that, as far as possible, the first reports shall cover all who have died in our hands at any previous time.

"Blanks for making the reports will be furnished from this office.

"Very respectfully,
"Your obedient servant,
(Signed) "W. HOFFMAN,
"*Col. 3d Inf'y, Com.-Gen'l of Prisoners.*

"Col. J. K. BARNES,
"*Inspector-General, U. S. A.,*
"*Acting Surgeon-General,*
"*Washington, D. C.*"

In compliance with the above request of the "Commissary-General of Prisoners," the report asked for will be furnished to him by Surgeons in charge of Hospitals where Prisoners of War are held, on the fifteenth and last days of each month.

By order of the Acting Surgeon General:

C. H. CRANE,
Surgeon, U. S. A.

CIRCULAR No. 24.

Surgeon-General's Office,
Washington, D.C., *November* 5, 1863.

To obviate the frequent discrepancies and contradictions occurring in "Certificates of Disability for Discharge," and those of Examining Surgeons for the Pension Bureau, hereafter Certificates of Disability will state *all* the causes of disability, where more than one exists, and the Medical Certificate will, in every instance, be made out in the handwriting of the Surgeon signing it.

By order of the Acting Surgeon-General:

C. H. CRANE,
Surgeon, U. S. A.

CIRCULAR No. 25.—GENERAL ORDERS No. 355.

War Department, Adjutant-General's Office,
Washington, *November* 4, 1863.

Medical Directors of Armies in the field will forward, direct to the Surgeon-General, at Washington, duplicates of their reports to their several Commanding Generals of the killed and wounded, after every engagement.

By order of the Secretary of War:

(Signed) E. D. TOWNSEND,
Assistant Adjutant-General.

Surgeon-General's Office,
Washington, D.C., *November* 11, 1863.

To carry out the intentions of the above Order, Medical Directors of Armies in the field will detail suitable officers, who will, under their instructions, collate and prepare for transmission to this office all obtainable statistics and data in connexion with past and future operations of those armies, which may be essential or useful in the accurate compilation of the Medical and Surgical history of the War. Particular attention is called to the following points:

The morale and sanitary condition of the troops, condition and amount of Medical and Hospital supplies, tents, ambulances, etc.; the point at or near the field where the wounded were attended to; degree of exposure of wounded to wet, cold, or heat; adequacy of supplies of water, food, stimulants, etc.; mode of removal of wounded from field to field hospitals; to what General Hospitals the wounded were transferred—by what means and where; the character and duration of the action, nature of wounds received, etc. When practicable, separate casualty lists will be made of commissioned officers, non-commissioned officers, and privates.

The attention of all Medical Officers is earnestly directed to the importance of this subject; without their coöperation no reliable record can be preserved—the vast experience of the past will remain with individuals, and be lost to the service and the country.

Jos. K. Barnes,
Medical Inspector-General,
Acting Surgeon-General.

CIRCULAR NO. 26.

Surgeon-General's Office,
Washington, D.C., *November* 24, 1863.

The attention of Medical Officers in charge of U. S. A. General Hospitals is invited to the importance of preparing illustrations of the results of surgical operations. These can in many instances be conveniently obtained by means of plaster casts, which are readily made without subjecting patients to the slightest inconvenience.

The casts most desired are those of stumps of amputation of every variety, and models of limbs upon which excisions may have been performed.

In selecting proper subjects for representation, it would be well to choose not only cases in which the results have been favorable, but also those in which they may have been unfavorable. In a collection like the National Museum, truthful representations of both good and bad results are alike instructive and valuable for future reference and study.

These casts, when made, should be forwarded to the Army Medical Museum by express. The expressage will be paid in Washington. All preparations should be accompanied by proper histories, with name, rank, and station of the contributor, who will be duly credited in the Museum Catalogue.

Jos. K. Barnes,
Acting Surgeon-General.

Surgeon-General's Office,
March 23, 1863.

The following instructions are for the information of those Surgeons to whom the "Army Microscope" is issued:

The microscope is to be kept carefully in a dry place, as free from dust as possible. When not in use, it is to be locked in its box, to protect it from dust, and to prevent its being handled by improper persons. Each objective to be preserved in its brass case.

In manipulating, the greatest pains must be taken not to injure or break the apparatus by hasty or inconsiderate movements. This is especially necessary in the use of the one-fifth of an inch objective, which, by carelessness in the adjustment of focus, may be crushed against the covering glass of the object, and in the preservation of the stage micrometer, which, resembling very closely an ordinary glass slip, is readily lost or broken, if not made the subject of peculiar care.

To clean the glasses of the eye-piece, it is usually sufficient to dust them off with a camel's hair pencil. Should the dust adhere, however, the glasses may be taken apart and wiped thoroughly, but gently, with a piece of soft old cambric. A new and perfectly clean chamois skin will answer the same purpose, but one that has been used for cleaning instruments, or any similar purpose, will not answer, as it is liable to contain gritty particles, which would scratch the glasses.

The dust specks seen in the field of the microscope are usually due to particles on the eye-piece, as can always be told by rotating it, when, of course, the specks will rotate with it, unless they are on the objective, in which case they will remain stationary.

The glasses of the objective may be cleaned in the same manner, but it is, as a general rule, unnecessary to take them apart for this purpose, the bottom glass only being likely to become soiled even in the course of years of careful use.

Volatile chemicals, such as ammonia, nitric and hydrochloric acids, sulphuretted hydrogen, and the like, are not to be kept in the same room with the microscope, the glasses and brass-work of which they injuriously attack.

In the examination of urine, and in the use of reagents, pains are to be taken not to soil the brass-work of the instrument, which, in careful hands, should not tarnish even in several years.

The one-fifth of an inch objective being adjusted for the examination of objects covered with a thin glass cover, cannot be advantageously used without this precaution. Especially is this cover essential in the examination of blood and urine, which, if not thus protected, are liable to soil and injure the bottom glass of the objective.

W. A. HAMMOND,
Surgeon-General.

CIRCULAR NO. 1.

Surgeon-General's Office,
Washington, D.C., *January* 18, 1864.

By a decision of the First Assistant Postmaster-General, "Hospital Stewards and Medical Cadets have no right to frank letters to any Department. Their reports should be made through the Surgeon in charge of the hospital, or the Commanding Officer of the Post where they are stationed."

JOS. K. BARNES,
Acting Surgeon-General.

CIRCULAR NO. 2.

Surgeon-General's Office,
Washington, D.C., *January* 19, 1864.

The attention of Medical Officers in charge of U. S. Hospitals is called to the imperative necessity for more strict compliance with Paragraph 1286, Revised Army Regulations, 1863, regarding Descriptive Lists of soldiers leaving hospitals. Whether a soldier be transferred from one hospital to another, to his regiment, or to any other point, his complete and certified Descriptive List must be at once transmitted to the proper officer.

Hereafter, failure to comply with this regulation will be considered disobedience of orders, and as such reported to the Secretary of War for his action.

JOS. K. BARNES,
Acting Surgeon-General.

CIRCULAR NO. 3.

Surgeon-General's Office,
Washington, D.C., *January* 26, 1864.

By order of the Secretary of War, gratuitous issue of necessary clothing will be made to soldiers returning to duty from Small-Pox Hospitals.

JOS. K. BARNES,
Acting Surgeon-General.

CIRCULAR NO. 4.

Surgeon-General's Office,
Washington, D.C., *February* 19, 1864.

I.—Separate reports of sick and wounded rebel prisoners of war, treated in U. S. General or Post Hospitals, will be made monthly to this office.

II.—Whenever white and colored troops are treated in the same hospital (either General or Post), separate reports of sick and wounded will be made, in order that the sickness and mortality rates of each race can be correctly ascertained.

III.—Monthly Sick Reports from regiments or detachments of colored troops will present on the first page of the report the number of sick of enlisted men only; the names, rank, and diseases of sick officers of these regiments will be placed under the head of Remarks.

JOS. K. BARNES,
Acting-Surgeon-General.

CIRCULAR NO. 5.

Surgeon-General's Office,
Washington, D.C., *March* 1, 1864.

Surgeons in charge of General Hospitals are hereby positively instructed that when a soldier is discharged from service on account of *wounds received in action*, that fact will be entered both on the discharge and final statement of the soldier.

JOS. K. BARNES,
Acting Surgeon-General.

CIRCULAR NO. 7.

Snrgeon-General's Office,
Washington, D.C., *April* 7, 1864.

The following regulations relative to Hospital Stewards are published for the information of all concerned:

I.—Persons desiring the appointment of Hospital Steward will make application in their own handwriting, to the Surgeon-General of the Army, Washington, D.C., or Assistant-Surgeon-General at Louisville, Ky., accompanied by one or more testimonials from respectable persons as to their good moral character, and competency as druggists. If the applicant be a soldier, the application must be forwarded through the Medical Director of the Department or Army in which he is serving, who will endorse the same; if sent through any other channel (under these circumstances), it will be disapproved.

II.—If the application is favorably considered, the candidate will receive a permit to present himself before the nearest Army Medical Board, or, if there is none in session within a convenient distance, to the nearest Medical Director, who will convene one, to consist of three Medical Officers, who will rigidly scrutinize the moral character and physical qualifications of the candidate, and examine him as to fitness for this position, recommending no person for appointment who does not possess a fair English education and a sufficient knowledge of pharmacy to enable him to take charge of the dispensing department of a General Hospital. The Board will report the result of each examination to this office, or the Assistant-Surgeon-General's. If the Board has been convened by a Medical Director, in case of a favorable report, he will endorse thereon, for the information of the Surgeon-General, whether the services of such approved applicants are required in his Department. The Assistant-Surgeon-General will forward all reports received by him to this office, with such recommendation in each case as he may deem proper.

III.—Applicants must be between the ages of twenty-one and forty-five, and of sound physical constitution.

IV.—Hospital Stewards are enlisted for the period of *three* years, and are entitled to thirty dollars per month, and such bounty, clothing, and rations as are allowed to other enlisted men.

JOS. K. BARNES,
Acting Surgeon-General.

CIRCULAR LETTER.

Surgeon-General's Office,
Washington, D.C., *January* 14, 1864.

The Board of Medical Officers assembled at the city of Philadelphia for the purpose of examining the different models submitted to them for an artificial arm, having reported in favor of Selpho's model for cases of amputation below, and the Lincoln model above the elbow joint, you are authorized to order artificial arms from these manufacturers, for soldiers who may be entitled to receive them, under the same instructions as heretofore printed for artificial limbs, the price not to exceed fifty dollars ($50.00).

In compliance with the recommendation of the Board, when a soldier may desire to purchase "the more elegant and expensive arm of Palmer," fifty dollars will be allowed towards payment for the same, upon a written application to that effect to a Medical Director, who will satisfy himself that the transaction has been carried out in good faith.

By order of the Acting Surgeon-General:

C. H. CRANE,
Surgeon, U. S. A.

CIRCULAR LETTER.

Surgeon-General's Office,
Washington, D.C., *January* 15, 1864.

SIR: You will immediately communicate to this office the probable amount of ice that will be required for General Hospitals within your Department to December 1st, 1864; the present facilities for proper storage and preservation; the points at which it can be most advantageously delivered; and such other information as will be useful in making the awards of contracts.

By order of the Acting Surgeon-General:

C. H. CRANE,
Surgeon, U. S. A.

Medical Director,

CIRCULAR LETTER.

Surgeon-General's Office,
Washington, D.C., *January* 20, 1864.

SIR: Hereafter, you are directed to transmit to this office, regularly, copies of your Weekly consolidated Sick Reports, as soon as possible after they are received by you. You will also cause copies of any Weekly Sick Reports of the Army under your direction, for the past, which may be on file in your office, to be forwarded to the Surgeon-General as soon as convenient.

By order of the Acting Surgeon-General:

C. H. CRANE,
Surgeon, U. S. A.

Medical Director,

CIRCULAR LETTER.

Surgeon-General's Office,
Washington, D.C., *January* 22, 1864.

Your attention is respectfully called to the fact that the requirements of Circular No. 3, S. G. O., of January 30th, 1863, are almost uniformly disregarded by Medical Officers, especially the directions contained in Paragraph 2d relative to the manner of accounting for certain non-perishable articles paid for from the Hospital Fund.

You will, therefore, at once instruct all Medical Officers in charge of hospitals under your jurisdiction to comply in future strictly with those orders.

By order of the Acting Surgeon-General:

C. H. CRANE,
Surgeon, U. S. A.

Medical Director,

CIRCULAR LETTER.

Surgeon-General's Office,
Washington, D.C., *January* 26, 1864.

SIR: Hereafter you are directed to transmit to this office, regularly, copies of your Weekly Consolidated Sick Reports, as soon as possible after they are received by you. You will also cause copies of any Weekly Sick Reports of the Army under your direction, for the past, which may be on file in your office, to be forwarded to the Surgeon-General as soon as convenient.

By order of the Acting Surgeon-General:

C. H. CRANE,
Surgeon, U. S. A.

Medical Director,

CIRCULAR LETTER.

Surgeon-General's Office,
Washington, D.C., *January* 29, 1864.

[COPY.]

GENERAL ORDERS NO. 23.

War Department, Adjutant-General's Office,
Washington, D.C., *January* 16, 1864.

General Orders No. 390, dated War Department, Adjutant-General's Office, Washington, December 8, 1863, is hereby revoked, and the following substituted therefor:

The employment of persons of African descent, male or female as cooks or nurses, will be permitted in all U. S. General Hospitals.

When so employed they will receive ten dollars per month and one ration. They will be paid by the nearest Medical Disbursing Officer, on rolls similar to those used in the payment of men of the Hospital Corps.

By order of the Secretary of War:

(Signed) E. D. TOWNSEND,
Assistant Adjutant-General.

Respectfully furnished for the information of Medical Directors.

By order of the Acting-Surgeon-General.

C. H CRANE,
Surgeon, U. S. A.

CIRCULAR LETTER.

Surgeon-General's Office,
Washington, *January* 30, 1864.

(EXTRACT.)

Quartermaster-General's Office,
Washington, *January* 23, 1864.

COL. J. C. BARNES.
Acting Surgeon-General:

* * * * * * * *

You are respectfully informed that the Hospital and Ambulance Flags, established in General Orders, No. 9 (current series), from the Adjutant-General's Office, will be furnished upon requisition by this Department.

Very respectfully, your obedient servant.

By Order of the Quartermaster-General:

ALEX. J. PERRY, *A. Q. M.*

Respectfully furnished for the information of Medical Directors and Purveyors.

By order of the Acting Surgeon-General:

C. H. CRANE,
Surgeon, U. S. A.

CIRCULAR LETTER.

Surgeon-General's Office,
Washington, D.C., *February* 1, 1864.

The Reports of Medical and Hospital Property received, issued, and remaining on hand at the different Purveying Depôts will, hereafter, be rendered monthly instead of semi-monthly as heretofore.

By Order of the Acting Surgeon-General:

C. H. CRANE.
Surgeon, U. S. A.

CIRCULAR LETTER.

Surgeon-General's Office,
Washington, D.C., *February* 4, 1854.

To Surgeon in charge of ——— Hospital:

SIR: Immediately upon the reception of this circular, you will fill up the appended blank and return the circular by mail directly to this office. Hereafter in all cases of small-pox or varioloid treated in your hospital, the fact of previous vaccination, re-vaccination, or the absence of either, will, when positively known, be entered on the Hospital Register, and the number of cases of each be reported in the Monthly Sick Report under the head of Remarks.

Very respectfully,

Your obedient servant:

By Order of the Acting Surgeon-General:

C. H. Crane,

Surgeon, U. S. A.

——— Hospital, ——— 186—	Small-Pox.		Varioloid.	
	Cases.	Deaths.	Cases.	Deaths.
Number of Patients treated in this hospital previous to January, 1864, of whom it is known whether they were previously vaccinated or not,				
Number positively known to have been vaccinated once successfully prior to the attack, ...				
Number positively known to have been successfully vaccinated more than once prior to the attack,....................................				

CIRCULAR LETTER.

Surgeon-General's Office,
Washington, D.C., *February* 6, 1864.

Ice provided from the appropriation for the Medical Department is exclusively for the use of the sick in General and Post Hospitals, and will not under any circumstances be issued or otherwise disposed of to officers or soldiers not actually under treatment in them. The most rigid economy must be observed in the issue and use of ice so supplied. Issues to hospitals will be made upon the estimate of one pound daily per patient at Washington and points south of it; half a pound daily per patient at all points north of Washington, which, with proper care, will be found an ample allowance. Medical Directors will give such orders as will insure compliance with these instructions.

Very respectfully,

Your obedient servant,

By order of the Acting Surgeon-General:

C. H. Crane,

Surgeon, U. S. Army.

CIRCULAR LETTER.

Surgeon-General's Office,
Washington, D.C., *February* 11, 1864.

The attention of Medical Directors is called to the frequency of discharges upon "Certificates of Disability," for "Disease of the Heart," and the necessity for a more stringent application of Paragraph 4, page 6, General Orders No. 212, War Department, Sept. 9, 1863.

Mere functional disturbance does not disqualify for active service, and such cases should be retained in hospital only long enough to establish a correct diagnosis. Organic disease of the heart, without grave constitutional implications, does not entitle to discharge, but may be sufficient cause for transfer to the Invalid Corps. In those well-marked and unmistakable cases, accompanied by constitutional symptoms, leaving no doubt of entire disability, which alone entitles to discharge, the certificate of the Surgeon must set forth these facts fully before receiving the approval of a Medical Director.

By order of the Acting Surgeon-General:

C. H. Crane,
Surgeon, U. S. Army.

Medical Director,

CIRCULAR LETTER.

Surgeon-General's Office,
Washington, D.C., *February* 12, 1864.

One copy of *Wood's Practice of Medicine* has been added to the present Standard Table of Field Supplies, and will hereafter be issued to regiments upon proper requisition.

By order of the Acting Surgeon-General:

C. H. Crane,
Surgeon, U. S. Army.

Medical Director,

CIRCULAR LETTER.

Surgeon-General's Office,
Washington, D.C., *February* 15, 1864.

The rendition of "Monthly Statements of Approved Requisitions varying from the Supply Table," called for in a letter from this office of August 4, 1863, will in future be discontinued, since the purposes for which they were required have been attained.

By order of the Acting-Surgeon-General:

C. H. Crane,
Surgeon, U. S. Army.

Medical Director,

CIRCULAR LETTER.

Surgeon-General's Office,
Washington, D.C., *February* 17, 1864.

I.—The attention of Medical Directors is called to the following decision of the Commissary-General of Subsistence:

"When cows have been purchased out of Hospital Fund, it is believed that the expense of forage therefor, and all other necessary expenses for the support and keeping of these cows, is a proper charge against Hospital Fund.

(Signed) "J. P. TAYLOR,
" *Com.-Gen'l Subsistence.*"

II.—Pension Claims are referred to this office for official evidence of cause of death in the cases of soldiers known to have died on hospital transports and trains, but of whom no report had been made to the Surgeon-General. Such information is required to secure the rights of widows and orphans of deceased soldiers, and Medical Directors will hereafter order all Medical Officers detailed on duty with the transportation of troops to report to them up n the termination of the voyage or journey, the name, rank, company, regiment, date, and cause of death, of every soldier who has died during the transfer. A certified copy of such report will be at once forwarded to this office.

By order of the Acting Surgeon-General:

C. H. CRANE,
Surgeon, U. S. Army.

Medical Director,.

CIRCULAR LETTER.

Surgeon-General's Office,
Washington, D.C., *March* 5, 1864.

War Department, Adjutant-General's Office,
Washington, *January* 22, 1864.

SIR: The following instructions from the Secretary of War are furnished for your information and guidance:

Upon the recommendation of the Acting Surgeon-General, permanently disabled soldiers, who are furloughed from various sections of the country, are permitted to report to the nearest Medical Directors, who are hereby authorized to place them in U. S. Hospitals until further action in their cases can be taken.

I have the honor to be, sir,
Very respectfully, your obedient servant,

(R. & R. R., No. 8.) *Asst. Adjutant-General.*

Respectfully furnished for the information of Medical Directors.

By order of the Acting Surgeon-General:

C. H. CRANE,
Surgeon, U. S. A.

MEMORANDA FOR THE USE OF MEDICAL PURVEYORS IN THE PREPARATION AND SETTLEMENT OF THEIR ACCOUNTS.

1. Money accounts, comprising an Account Current, an Abstract of Disbursements, and the necessary vouchers, are to be sent monthly to the Second Auditor of the Treasury within ten days after the end of each month. These accounts should include an Abstract of the several sums retained as an Internal Revenue Tax,

and the receipts of the proper officer for the money paid into the Treasury on that account. As tax receipts are now sent directly from the Bureau of Internal Revenue to the Surgeon-General's Office, accounts need not be delayed until such receipts reach the disbursing officer. Copies or duplicates should not be sent as vouchers, but in all cases the original bills, rolls, &c, with the receipts, endorsements, and approvals in virtue of which they were paid.

2. Duplicates of any of the foregoing papers are not necessary for the use of the Surgeon-General's Office, as the Auditor transmits packages of accounts unbroken to this office for examination.

3. The subject of Internal Revenue Tax should not be introduced into the Abstract of Disbursements or Account Current. A payment of a month's salary of $100 should be stated as $100 and not $98.50 The receipt, however, must be for the *nett* amount.

4. When a disbursing officer has funds pertaining to two or more appropriations, separate accounts should be rendered for each.

5. The Second Auditor requests that there may be transmitted to him, through this office, monthly statements of the Treasury Certificates paid on account of private physicians.

6. The Summary Statements of Funds heretofore made monthly are desired semi-monthly (observing the requirements of Section 4), with the addition of a note showing the estimated amount of outstanding bills.

7. Every Bill of purchase should be sent as soon as practicable to this Office to be examined and recorded. It should be accompanied by a corresponding property Receipt, or receipted Invoice, so marked and numbered that it may be used with facility in examining the Quarterly Property Return. The receipt will be retained to be so used, and no further duplicate or copy of it need be sent.

8. The Bill of purchase, when examined, recorded, and marked, will be promptly returned, whether paid or unpaid; except in cases where it is deemed advisable to send an unpaid account to the Treasury or elsewhere for settlement. Any corrections that may be necessary will be noted on the account when it is returned.

9. The Medical Purveyor will determine from the circumstances of each case how many shall be included in a single account; but it would seem to be much more convenient to include the purchase of a week, two weeks, or even a month, in a single account and property receipt than to make a multitude of small bills for the various articles bought of the same person.

10. When, at the end of a month, it is inconvenient to spare bills long enough to send them to this office before the monthly accounts are rendered, duplicates or copies need not be sent, nor should the rendering of the account be delayed. This office would rather wait until the monthly accounts arrive than examine and record copies. Yet even in this case the property invoices should be sent.

11. Property Returns are to be rendered to this office, quarterly and in duplicate, with Abstracts and vouchers for receipts and issues, which need not be sent in duplicate. The several columns of the Abstract should agree with the several invoices such as those named in Section 7, and should be marked with corresponding numbers. One general receipt for all property received during the quarter is not sufficient, on account of the great difficulty of verification.

12. When a disbursing officer is under bonds, the date of such bonds should be noted at the head of the Account Current immediately after the officer's name.

13. When alterations or additional vouchers are required, after the accounts of a disbursing officer have been examined by the Second Auditor, it is highly desirable that all such additional matter should be transmitted through this office, or a copy of the same be furnished.

Surgeon-General's Office,
March 7, 1864.

CIRCULAR LETTER.

Surgeon-General's Office,
Washington, D.C., *March* 7, 1864.

[COPY.]

War Department, Adjutant-General's Office,
Washington, *January* 22, 1864.

CIRCULAR No. 9.

The following instructions from the Secretary of War are furnished for the information and guidance of all concerned:

Officers signing the discharge papers of enlisted men who are discharged on Surgeon's Certificate of Disability, will note, on the back of the Discharge, where the conduct of the man has not been meritorious, as required by General Order, No. 212, of 1863, for admission into the Invalid Corps, that he is *not a proper person for the Invalid Corps.*

E. D. TOWNSEND,
Asst. Adjutant-General.

Respectfully furnished for the information of Medical Directors, Surgeons in Charge of General Hospitals, etc.

By order of the Acting Surgeon-General:

C. H. CRANE,
Surgeon, U. S. A.

CIRCULAR LETTER.

Surgeon-General's Office,
Washington, D.C., *March* 8, 1864.

[COPY.]

War Department, Adjutant-General's Office,
Washington, *February* 6, 1864.

CIRCULAR No. 18.

In future, each officer in charge of enlisted men absent from their Regiments will report at the end of every month, to the Regimental or Company Commanders of the men under their charge, whether they are sick, in confinement, in hospital, on detached service, etc.; their station, the duties which each man is performing, and the authority for detaining him, giving the number and date of the order. Also whether they are sick, or fit for service, and any other particulars about them which may be necessary for the information of their Commanding Officers in keeping a correct account of the pay, clothing, station, duties, etc., of each soldier. Without such reports, men cannot receive the pay actually due them.

E. D. Townsend,
Asst. Adjutant-General.

Respectfully furnished for the information of Medical Directors, Surgeons in Charge of General Hospitals, etc.

By order of the Acting Surgeon-General:

C. H. Crane,
Surgeon, U. S. A.

CIRCULAR LETTER.

Surgeon-General's Office,
Washington, D.C., *March* 9, 1864.

The directions conveyed in a Circular Letter from this office to Medical Purveyors, dated October 30, 1863, relative to the payment of contract physicians whose contracts have been terminated, are hereby revoked, and they will, in future, be paid upon the presentation of warrants from the Treasury, a certificate of non-indebtedness to the United States for medical and hospital property not being required.

Medical Directors will continue, however, to comply with the instructions contained in letter from Surgeon-General's office, December 22, 1863, by stating on each account whether the physician is at the time in service, and by giving the date of termination of contract when it has been annulled.

By order of the Acting Surgeon-General:

C. H. Crane,
Surgeon, U. S. A.

Surgeon-General's Office,
Washington, D.C., *March* 10, 1864.

Sir: The Reports of Wounded and of Surgical Operations for the months of October, November, and December, 1863, called for by Special Circular from the Acting Surgeon-General of December 26, 1863, have not as yet been received from the hospital under your charge.

I am instructed by the Acting Surgeon-General to request that you will cause these reports to be immediately prepared, and that you will then transmit them directly to this office.

Very respectfully,

Your obedient servant,

By order of the Acting Surgeon-General:

C. H. CRANE,

Surgeon, U. S. A.

Medical Officer in charge of ——
U. S. A. General Hospital.

CIRCULAR LETTER.

Surgeon-General's Office,
Washington, D.C., *March* 22, 1864.

GENERAL ORDERS NO. 107.

War Department, Adjutant-General's Office,
Washington, *March* 16, 1864.

CLOTHING OF SMALL-POX PATIENTS.

Hereafter, upon the discharge of soldiers from small-pox hospitals, the following articles of clothing will be issued to them gratuitously by the Quartermaster's Department:

1 pair Trowsers,
1 Blouse,
1 Shirt,
1 pair Drawers,
1 pair Socks,
1 Cap.

The infected clothing belonging to the men will be burned.

By order of the Secretary of War:

E. D. TOWNSEND,

Assistant Adjutant-General.

Respectfully furnished for the information of Medical Directors.

By order of the Acting Surgeon-General:

C. H. CRANE,

Surgeon, U. S. Army.

CIRCULAR LETTER.

Surgeon-General's Office,
Washington, D.C., *March* 23, 1864.

Medical Directors of armies in the field will issue the "Classified Return of Wounds and Injuries received in Action" to the chief Medical Officers of corps and divisions, who will see that they are properly distributed.

This form, correctly filled up by the senior Medical Officer of the command engaged, will be transmitted, in duplicate, through the proper channel, to the Medical Director of the army within three days after every action.

The Medical Director of the Army will, as soon as possible,

forward to the Surgeon-General a Consolidated Return of all Casualties, according to the same form. He will at the same time transmit one copy of all duplicate returns received from his subordinate Medical Officers.

JOS. K. BARNES,
Acting Surgeon-General.

CIRCULAR LETTER.

Surgeon-General's Office,
Washington, D.C., *March* 24, 1864.

All arrivals, transfers, discharges, desertions, and deaths of paroled prisoners in General Hospitals will be promptly reported to their regimental commanders.

By order of the Acting Surgeon-General:

C. H. CRANE,
Surgeon, U. S. Army.

CIRCULAR LETTER.

Surgeon-General's Office,
Washington, D.C., *March* 26, 1864.

The attention of Medical Directors is specially requested to the following points relative to the Contracts and Pay Accounts of Acting Assistant-Surgeons, errors and confusion having arisen on these subjects:

I.—Contracts with private physicians should be executed in triplicate; one copy to be retained by the physician, one kept on file in the office of his Medical Director, and the third immediately forwarded (approved) to the Surgeon-General, with usual post-office address of the person contracted with.

II.—Officers terminating these contracts should immediately notify this office of the date and cause of such action, and date of the contract. All notices and orders relative to Acting Assistant-Surgeons should give their names in full. Upon the termination of his contract, an Acting Assistant-Surgeon should turn over to his successor, or to a Medical Purveyor, all medical and hospital property for which he is responsible, and transmit returns and vouchers at once to this office. His accounts will be suspended until this is done.

III.—Accounts for medical services under contract must exhibit the following facts:

1. The place of service.

2. The dates between which the services were rendered. The Treasury Department assumes every month to be composed of thirty days, and accounts for fractional parts of two successive months must be so calculated; thus, from the 21st of August to the 10th of September, the calculation of time will be from the 21st to the 30th of August, inclusive (ignoring the 31st), ten

days, and from the 1st to the 10th of September, inclusive, ten days—making the time to be paid for twenty days.

3. The name of the hospital, camp, post, regiment, or command, in or with which the services were rendered.

4. The class of persons with whom rendered; whether U. S. forces, colored troops, prisoners of war, military prisoners, refugees, contrabands, or whether the services were rendered in Small-Pox Hospitals.

5. The date of the contract under which the services were rendered, and the name of the officer with whom the con ract was made.

6. If for service at a post, or with a detachment, the strength of the command must be stated.

IV.—Accounts must be made out for periods of one or more complete months, commencing with the date of entry upon service. No account embracing fractional periods of a month will receive attention, unless it appears upon the face thereof, either that the station of the physician has been changed or his contract annulled; but accounts for any length of time may be presented on one set of duplicates, subject only to the exemptions specified.

V.—Accounts for several months' service, if rendered separately, must be continuous; for the Treasury Department will not pay an account for one month until that of the preceding month has been settled.

VI.—Officers certifying to accounts of a "Private Physician under Contract," must give their official title, and state explicitly the capacity in which they are serving; otherwise their authority to make such a certificate may be questioned. E. g., A. B., Surgeon U. S. A., *in charge* ——— *General Hospital.* C. D., Surg. Vols., *Medical Director*, 1*st Division*, 2*d Army Corps.* E. F., Col. 40th Ohio Vols., *Commanding Post, Garrison, Regiment.* As they are also held personally responsible for the truth of every statement contained therein, certificates signed "By Order" or "For Medical Director" will be disregarded.

VII.—When medicines have been supplied at a percentage of the amount of compensation, a statement to the effect that they have been furnished as required must be added to the usual certificate of service, or the claim for medicines cannot be approved.

VII.—All accounts certified by other officers than a Medical Director must be forwarded to this office through that of the Medical Director of the Department in which the services were rendered, that he may endorse his knowledge of their correctness.

IX.—In all cases of absence from duty, the dates and cause of such absence must be clearly stated. If a substitute has been furnished, his name in full must be given, with a statement showing that he has sa isfactorily performed all the duties incumbent upon the contract physician.

X.—When instruments are furnished to a contract physician by a Medical Purveyor, the kind, and cost price thereof, are to be reported by the Medical Purveyor to this office. The cost price is then deducted from the first account for services rendered subsequent to such reports. The instruments then become the *private* property of the contract physician, and are in no case to be turned back to a Purveyor or other officer without the written order of this office.

XI.—Officers requiring medical attendance for their commands should, when practicable, apply to the nearest Medical Director, who will, if satisfied of its necessity, at once supply the required aid, or authorize such action as the interests of the service may demand. When the necessity for immediate medical attendance is great, and the service would suffer by delay, the officer in command will employ a private physician, by contract or otherwise, as provided in Revised Army Regulations, and he will notify the Medical Director of the Department of the facts, sending him two copies of the contract for approval.

By order of the Acting Surgeon-General:

C. H. CRANE,
Surgeon, U. S. Army.

CIRCULAR LETTER.

Surgeon-General's Office,
Washington, D.C., *March* 28, 1864.

SIR: You are hereby directed to fill up the accompanying "Report of Wounded" and "Report of Surgical Operations" for the months of January, February, and March, 1864.

The *Report of Wounded* will consist of an accurate and legible copy of all cases of wounded entered on the Hospital Register during the quarter.

The *Report of Surgical Operations* will consist of a correct copy of the Register of Surgical Operations for the same period.

A list of wounded *remaining* under treatment on the 31st December, 1863, in the hospital under your charge, and *on furlough*, is inclosed—you are directed to fill up the column, "Result and Date," opposite the respective names.

Additional details for the present quarter of "Surgical Operations remaining under Treatment, December 31, 1863," you will report on *appended* slips of paper.

Blank sets of reports on secondary hæmorrhage, tetanus, and pyæmia, are also inclosed. These you will fill up in the usual manner. Should no such cases have occurred in the hospital under your charge during the time specified, you will so state in your letter of transmission.

All of the reports above alluded to will, when compiled, be forwarded directly to the Acting Surgeon-General.

By order of the Acting Surgeon-General:

C. H. CRANE,
Surgeon, U. S. A.

To the Medical Officer in charge
——————— *U. S. A. General Hospital.*

CIRCULAR LETTER.

Surgeon-General's Office,
Washington, D.C., *March* 31, 1864.

SIR: You will instruct Surgeons in Charge of Hospitals under your control to turn in to Medical Purveyors those bottles, jars, pots, and canisters *only* that have been issued from Purveying Depôts and remain fit for re-issue.

By order of the Acting Surgeon-General:

C. H. CRANE,
Surgeon, U. S. A.

Medical Director.

CIRCULAR LETTER.

Surgeon-General's Office,
Washington, D.C., *April* 22, 1864.

The following Order from the War Department is respectfully furnished for your information and guidance.

By order of the Acting Surgeon-General:

C. H. CRANE,
Surgeon, U. S. A.

GENERAL ORDERS No. 127.

War Department, Adjutant-General's Office,
Washington, *March* 29, 1864.

I.—Medical Directors of Departments will establish a General Hospital, at some convenient point within their respective Departments, for the reception and treatment of sick and wounded officers, but no expenditures for the construction of new hospitals for this purpose will be incurred without special authority. They will detail a Surgeon-in-Charge, who will make requisitions upon the Medical Purveyor for medicines, hospital stores, furniture, etc., according to the standard Supply Table of the Medical Department, and will hire the nurses, cooks, and laundresses required. Hospital Stewards assigned to Officers' General Hospitals will be paid on the regular muster and pay rolls.

II.—On the recommendation of the Medical Director of the Department, a commissioned medical officer will be detailed to act permanently as Treasurer for each Officers' General Hospital, who shall not be removed without sufficient cause. The Treasurer shall have the custody of the funds of the Hospital, and shall perform such duties in relation to collecting, disbursing, and accounting for the same, and such other duties as may be prescribed by the Surgeon-General.

III.—On the last day of each calendar month, and immediately on leaving the Hospital, by return to duty, furlough, or otherwise, each officer shall pay to the Treasurer the sum of one dollar for each and every day he has been in the Hospital, and for which he has not already paid as herein provided. When an officer has employed a special attendant, he shall pay thirty cents a day additional for each day such attendant was subsisted in the Hospital. Company officers of volunteers, while in such Officers' General Hospital, shall be considered as "on detached service without troops," for the purpose of drawing their pay and settling their indebtedness to the Hospital, and may be paid on separate pay accounts, instead of on the muster and pay rolls.

IV.—When an officer is not provided with money, and is unable to obtain it, he will give a certificate of indebtedness, in triplicate, to the Treasurer of the Hospital, in such form as shall be prescribed by the Surgeon-General,* for the amount due from him to the Hospital. The Treasurer shall immediately forward, for stoppage, two copies of the certificate to the Chief Paymaster of the Pay District in which the Hospital may be located, retaining the remaining copy for his own reference and security. When an officer is discharged from the Hospital to return to a regiment serving beyond the limits of the Pay District in which such Hospital is located, the Treasurer shall forward the certificates of indebtedness which the officer may have given to the proper Chief Paymaster, if known to him; otherwise, to the Paymaster General, for such reference.

V.—The Chief Paymaster of the Pay District will immediately cause the certificates of indebtedness to be placed in the hands of the Paymaster of the Hospital (or of the regiment, should the officer have left the Hospital), with instructions to stop the amounts of the first payment of the officers by whom the certificates were given. The Paymaster will take the receipt of each officer for the full amount of his pay account, and transmit the deducted sums to the Treasurer of the Hospital to which they are

---

* FORM OF A TRIPLICATE RECEIPT.

.... Officers' Hospital,

............186..

I HEREBY CERTIFY *that there is due from me to the............Hospital,*
For.......days' board from.......to.......inclusive $......
For.......days' subsistence of servant .... $......

$......

[TRIPLICATE.]

I CERTIFY *that the sum of.....................stated above is the total amount due this Hospital from.......................remaining to be accounted for.*

OFFICERS' HOSPITAL, *Treasurer......Hospital.*

due, who will endorse receipt therefor upon the duplicate certificates in the Paymaster's hands, or furnish duplicate abstracts of receipts signed by him, and embracing in one receipt the names of all the officers on whose accounts the sums have been remitted. The Paymaster will also forward monthly an abstract of certificates thus paid to the Surgeon-General.

VI.—Officers of the Subsistence Department will make *separate* abstracts of the sales to each Officers' General Hospital during each calendar month, and will report the same to the Commissary-General of Subsistence in the manner provided by regulations in relation to sales to officers. Payment for stores thus purchased of the Subsistence Department shall be made by the Treasurer monthly, and in cash, when practicable; but when the Treasurer has not money on hand sufficient to liquidate the entire indebtedness of the Hospital to the Subsistence Department, he shall give to the Commissary accountable for the stores sold a certificate of indebtedness, in duplicate, for the amount remaining unpaid, which certificate shall be a valid claim against the Hospital, and be paid from the first moneys received thereafter by the Treasurer, and until paid shall be considered as a sufficient cash voucher to the Commissary for the amount stated therein. When the Treasurer pays this certificate of indebtedness he shall take the receipt of the Commissary for the amount thus paid him, and shall report his action in this matter to the Commissary General of Subsistence, stating the date and amount of each certificate thus cancelled, the name of the Commissary receiving the money therefor, etc.

VII.—Medical Directors of Armies in the field, when necessary, will establish temporary Hospitals in the rear of such armies, to be governed by the above regulations. Medical Directors of Armies and of Departments and Medical Inspectors will frequently inspect Officers' General Hospitals, and in addition to the usual course of hospital inspection, they will investigate the manner in which the Treasurer performs his duties, and promptly report any neglect on his part to the Surgeon-General.

VIII.—No officer whose certificate of indebtedness to a Hospital remains unpaid by him shall receive pay without deducting therefrom the amount of this indebtedness and leaving it in the hands of the Paymaster, who shall give him duplicate receipts therefor, one of which the officer shall immediately forward to the Treasurer of the Hospital for which the stoppage is made. A violation of this paragraph will subject the officer so offending to court-martial for disobedience of orders.

IX.—When an officer dies in Hospital, the Treasurer shall immediately ascertain the amount of his indebtedness to the Hospital, and prepare an account thereof in triplicate, which shall be certified to be correct by both the Treasurer and the Surgeon-in-Charge. One copy of this account shall be retained by the Treasurer, and the remaining two copies be forwarded to the Second Auditor of the Treasury, in order that, upon the final settlement of the officer's accounts, the amount of his indebtedness may be deducted from any pay due him, and remitted to the Treasurer of the Hospital.

By order of the Secretary of War:

E. D. TOWNSEND,
Assistant Adjutant-General.

CIRCULAR LETTER.

Surgeon-General's Office,
Washington, D.C., *April* 27, 1864.

[COPY.]

GENERAL ORDERS No. 129.

War Department, Adjutant-General's Office,
Washington, *March* 30, 1864.

The attention of all officers is called to the Army Regulations and General Orders in regard to correspondence on official matters. All such correspondence must be conducted through the proper official channels, except in cases of pressing necessity, which do not leave time for regular communication, and then the necessity must be stated. All applications or correspondence, through whomsoever made, in violation of this order, will not be responded to, and the writers will be arrested and tried for disobedience of orders, or recommended to the President for dismissal.

By Command of Lieutenant-General Grant:

E. D. TOWNSEND,
Assistant Adjutant-General.

The attention of all Medical Officers of the Army is called to the above order from the War Department, and a strict compliance with the same is enjoined.

By order of the Acting Surgeon-General:

C. H. CRANE,
Surgeon, U. S. Army.

CIRCULAR LETTER.

Surgeon-General's Office,
Washington, D.C., *May* 3, 1864.

In future the retention of $2.00 from the monthly pay of contract nurses will be discontinued, and the pay proper, $13.00, will be given each month.

The total retained pay that may be due these nurses will be stated upon the first muster-roll made after the receipt of this order, and will be paid by Medical Purveyors upon the duplicate certificate of Medical Officers in charge of hospital, which will be a sufficient voucher.

Very respectfully,
Your obedient servant,

By order of the Surgeon-General:

C. H. CRANE,
Surgeon, U. S. Army.

CIRCULAR LETTER.

Surgeon-General's Office,
Washington, D.C., *May* 26, 1864.

The following order from the War Department is respectfully furnished for your information and guidance:

War Department,
Washington, *May* 20, 1864.

Accounts for newspaper advertising for the Bureaus of the War Department must be rendered in duplicate, and state upon their face—

The name of the publisher or firm;

The name of the newspaper and the place where published;

The dates between which inserted;

The amount of matter and number of insertions charged for, and rate per square or line;

And must be accompanied by a full schedule of the customary advertising terms of the newspaper, unless the same shall have been previously filed with the Assistant Secretary of War.

Accounts must then be verified by the officer by whom the advertisements are signed, stating that the publication was authorized by him, and the number of insertions ordered.

Advertisements copied from other papers, *without authority,* will not be paid for.

The attention of officers is directed to the fact that the practice of ordering advertisements to be inserted "till day" of sale, etc., involves a useless expenditure, in cases where the station of the officer is remote from the place of publication.

Officers issuing advertisements for publication, will, at the same time, transmit copies of the same to the Assistant Secretary of War, stating the newspapers in which they are to be published, and the number of insertions ordered; and whenever only a portion of the official newspapers in any locality are selected to publish any advertisement, the officer will state his reasons for selecting the particular papers in question, and also his reasons for not advertising in the other official papers in that locality.

By order of the Secretary of War:

(Signed) C. A. Dana,
Assistant Secretary of War.

By order of the Acting Surgeon-General:

C. H. Crane,
Surgeon, U. S. A.

CIRCULAR LETTER.

Surgeon-General's Office,
Washington, D.C., *June* 1, 1864.

General Orders No. 191, of May 7th, 1864, declare all prisoners of war of the Federal Army, on parole at that date, exchanged; and, at the request of the Commissary-General of Prisoners,

Surgeons in Charge are directed to take up on the same rolls as other soldiers, all paroled prisoners who were in any of the United States General Hospitals at the date of the General Order, and report them to Colonel Hoffman, Commissary-General of Prisoners of War, as so transferred.

By order of the Acting Surgeon-General:

C. H. CRANE,
Surgeon, U. S. A.

CIRCULAR LETTER.

Surgeon-General's Office,
Washington, D.C., *June* 4, 1864.

The following Circular from the War Department is respectfully furnished for your information and guidance:

CIRCULAR NO. 41.

War Department, Adjutant-General's Office,
Washington, *May* 25, 1864.

1. The Secretary of War directs that, in cases where officers and enlisted men (such as exchanged prisoners, convalescents, etc.) are to be sent to their regiments in the field, they shall not be forwarded, unless it is probable that they will reach their regiments in time to serve at least ten days before the expiration of their term of service.

2. The attention of all commanders is invited to the orders from this office, directing that the men whose terms of service expire at the expiration of the original term of the regiment, should be sent to the State to which the regiment belongs, to be mustered out under the superintendence of the Chief Mustering Officer of the State. When the term of service of enlis ed men expires at other times, they should be mustered out of service by the Commissary or Assistant Commissary of Musters of the command in which they may be serving. When enlisted men are too sick to travel to the proper place of muster-out, they will be discharged for disability in the usual way, stating in addition the fact that the soldier's term of service has expired. The discharge of men of the Veteran Reserve Corps is provided for by Circular No. 12, current series, from this office.

E. D. TOWNSEND,
Assistant Adjutant-General.

By order of the Acting Surgeon-General:

C. H. CRANE,
Surgeon, U. S. A.

CIRCULAR LETTER.

Surgeon-General's Office,
Washington, D.C., *June* 13, 1864.

To facilitate the arrest of deserters from U. S. Army General Hospitals, the Surgeon in charge, as soon as a desertion is ascertained, will report the fact direct (and with copy of descriptive list) to the Provost-Marshal of the district in which the hospital is located, and to such other Provost-Marshals as might be of immediate aid in making the arrest.

This in addition to the Regular Reports of Deserters sent to the Provost-Marshal-General's Bureau.

By order of the Acting Surgeon-General:

C. H. CRANE,
Surgeon, U. S. A.

CIRCULAR LETTER.

**Surgeon-General's Office,
Washington, D.C., *June* 14, 1864.**

The following extracts from a Circular issued by the Commissary-General of Prisoners are published for the information of all Medical Officers concerned.

CIRCULAR.

**Office of Commissary-General of Prisoners,
Washington, D.C, *April* 20, 1864.**

III.—The hospital at depôts of prisoners of war will be under the immediate charge of the senior Medical Officer present, who will be held responsible to the Commanding Officer for its good order and the proper treatment of the sick. A fund for this hospital will be created as for other hospitals. It will be kept separate from the fund of the hospital for the troops, and will be expended for the objects specified, and in the manner prescribed in paragraph 1212, Revised Regulations for the Army, of 1863, except that the requisition of the Medical Officer in charge, and the bill of purchase, before payment, shall be approved by the Commanding Officer. When this "fund" is sufficiently large, it may be expended also for shirts and drawers for the sick, the expense of washing clothes, articles for policing purposes, and all articles and objects indispensably necessary to promote the sanitary condition of the hospital.

IV.—Surgeons in charge of hospitals where there are Prisoners of War will make the Commissary-General of Prisoners, through the Commanding Officer, semi-monthly reports of deaths, giving names, rank, regiment, and company; date and place of capture· date and cause of death; place of interment, and No. of grave. Effects of deceased prisoners will be taken possession of by the Commanding Officer, the money and valuables to be reported to this office (see note on blank reports), the clothing of any value to be given to such prisoners as require it. Money left by deceased prisoners, or accruing from the sale of their effects, will be placed in the Prison Fund.

The ration for issue to prisoners will be composed as follows:

Pork or Bacon,	10 oz.	(in lieu of Fresh Beef.)	
Fresh Beef,	14 do.		
Flour, or Soft Bread,	16 do.		
Hard Bread,	14 do.	(in lieu of Flour or Soft Bread.)	
Corn Meal,	16 do.	(in lieu of Flour or Bread.)	
Beans, or Peas,	12½ lbs.		to 100 rations.
Or Rice, or Hominy,	8 do.		to 100 rations.
Soap,	4 do.		to 100 rations.
Vinegar,	3 qts.		to 100 rations.
Salt,	3¾ lbs.		to 100 rations.
Potatoes,	15 do.		to 100 rations.

Sugar and coffee, or tea, will be issued only to the sick or wounded, on the recommendation of the Surgeon in charge, at the rate of twelve (12) pounds of sugar, five (5) pounds of ground or seven (7) pounds of green coffee, or one (1) pound of tea to the one hundred rations. This part of the ration will be allowed only for every other day.

The difference between the ration as above established, and the ration allowed by law to soldiers of the U. S. Army, constitutes the "savings" from which is formed the "Prison Fund."

VIII.—The Prison Fund is a credit with the Subsistence Department, and, at the request of the Commissary-General of Prisoners, may be transferred by the Commissary-General of Subsistence in manner prescribed by existing regulations for the transfer of Hospital Fund.

XVI.—When prisoners are seriously ill, their nearest relatives, being loyal, may be permitted to make them short visits; but under no other circumstances will visitors be admitted without the authority of the Commissary-General of Prisoners. At those places where the guard is inside the inclosure, persons having official business to transact with the Commander or other officer, will be admitted for such purposes, but will not be allowed to have any communication with prisoners.

By order of the Acting Surgeon-General:

C. H. CRANE,
Surgeon, U. S. A.

CIRCULAR LETTER.

Surgeon-General's Office,
Washington, D.C., *June* 15, 1864.

By authority of the Hon. Secretary of War, on and after July 1, 1864, the pay and allowances of hospital employés will be as follows, viz.:

I.—Male nurses and cooks (white), twenty-four ($24) dollars per month, and one ration per day.

II.—* * * * * Cooks (white), sixty (60) cents per day, and one ration.

III.—No clothing will be furnished, nor will any part of the monthly pay be retained.

IV.—All existing contracts will be annulled on July 1, prox.; the commutation value of clothing due will be paid, and new contracts entered upon at the rates above indicated.

Surgeons in charge of U. S. A. General Hospitals will not employ civilians as nurses (male) or cooks (male or female) without the approval of Medical Directors.

The application for permission to employ such persons must, in every instance, set forth the absolute necessity for their services, and the fact that it is impossible to procure suitable enlisted men for this duty.

Female nurses will be appointed under the provision of General Order No. 351, dated War Department, Adjutant-General's Office, Washington, October 29, 1863.

By order of the Acting Surgeon-General:

C. H. Crane,
Surgeon, U. S. A.

CIRCULAR LETTER.

Surgeon-General's Office,
Washington, D.C., *June* 22, 1864.

Surgeon D. L. Magruder, U. S. Army, Medical Purveyor, Louisville, Kentucky, is hereby appointed *Chief Medical Purveyor* for the Military Departments of the Ohio, Cumberland, Tennessee, Arkansas, Missouri, Kansas, the Northern and North-Western Departments.

All Medical Purveyors, and Medical Storekeepers acting as such, in the above-named Departments, will transmit to Surgeon Magruder, on the last day of each month, certified invoices of property remaining "on hand," and will obey such instructions and orders as he may deem proper to give them from time to time.

By order of the Surgeon-General:

C. H. Crane,
Surgeon, U. S. Army.

CIRCULAR LETTER.

Surgeon-General's Office,
Washington, D.C., *June* 24, 1864.

Medical Officers in charge of Hospitals are directed diligently to collect and preserve for the Army Medical Museum all pathological surgical specimens which may occur in the hospitals under their charge.

The objects which it is desired to collect for the Museum may be thus enumerated:

Fractures, compound and simple—fractures of the cranium.

Excised portions of bone.

Diseased bones and joints.

Exfoliations, especially those occurring in *stumps*.

Specimens illustrative of the structure of stumps (obliterated arteries, bulbous nerves, rounded bones, etc.).

Integumental wounds of entrance and of exit, from both the round and conoidal ball.

Wounds of vessels and nerves.

Vessels obtained subsequent to ligation and to secondary hæmorrhage.

Wounded viscera.

Photographic representations of extraordinary injuries, portraying the results of wounds, operations, or peculiar amputations.

Models of novel surgical appliances, and photographic views of new plans of dressing.

Plaster casts of stumps of amputations, and models of limbs upon which excisions may have been performed.

It is not intended to impose on medical officers the labor of dissecting and preparing the specimens they may contribute to the Museum. This will be done under the superintendence of the Curator.

In forwarding such pathological objects as compound fractures, bony specimens, and wet preparations generally, obtained after amputation, operation, or cadaveric examination, all unnecessary soft parts should first be roughly removed. Every specimen should then be wrapped separately in a cloth, so as to preserve all spicula and fragments. A small block of wood should be attached, with the name of the patient, the number of the specimen, and he name of the medical officer sending it inscribed in lead pencil. The inscription will be uninjured by the contact of fluids. The preparation should be then immersed in diluted alcohol or whiskey, contained in a keg or small cask. When a sufficient number of objects shall have accumulated, the cask should be forwarded directly to the Surgeon-General's office. The expenses of expressage will be defrayed in Washington. The receipt of the keg or package will be duly acknowledged by the Curator of the Museum.

In every instance, a corresponding list or history of the cases should, *at the same time*, be forwarded to this office. In this list the number and nature of every specimen should be clearly specified, and, when possible, its history should be given. The numbers attached to the specimens themselves, and the numbers in the list forwarded, should always correspond, and should be accompanied by the name and rank of the medical officer by whom sent. Every specimen will be duly credited in the Catalogue to the medical officer contributing it.

JOS. K. BARNES,
Acting Surgeon-General.

NOTE.—The following Medical Officers have been authorized to collect and forward specimens to the Museum from the localities in which they are respectively stationed:

Surgeon Lavington Quick, U.S.V., Baltimore.

Acting Assistant-Surgeon George Shrady, U.S.A., New York.

Surgeon Wm. Clendenin, U.S.V., Nashville.

Acting Assistant-Surgeon L. K. Baldwin, U.S.A., Philadelphia.
Surgeon M. Goldsmith, U.S.V., Louisville.
Assistant-Surgeon P. S. Connor, U.S.A., New Orleans.
Surgeon C. J. Kipp, U.S.V., Indianapolis.

To the Medical Officer in charge
——— ——— U. S. A. General Hospital.

CIRCULAR LETTER.

Surgeon-General's Office,
Washington, D.C., *June* 27, 1864.

Whenever a General Hospital is discontinued, the Medical Officer in charge will be instructed by the Medical Director of the Department to forward to the Surgeon-General's Office full reports of Wounded, Surgical Operations, Secondary Hæmorrhage, Tetanus, and Pyæmia, for the period of time elapsing between the *last quarterly* report and the date of *discontinuance* of the Hospital.

In the Reports of Wounded, and of Surgical Operations, especial care should be observed to furnish the results of those cases "remaining under treatment" at the date of the last quarterly report. A list of such cases can be obtained on application at the Surgeon-General's Office.

By order of the Acting Surgeon-General:

C. H. Crane,
Surgeon, U. S. A.

To Medical Director

INDEX.

perament; movement; specific gravity; dimensions; connections; special characters.—Information obtained by the ear.—Auscultation and percussion in surgery.—Information obtained by smell.—Information obtained by taste.—Circulatory, Respiratory, Nervous, Digestive, and Genito-Urinary systems.—Instruments employed in the investigation of surgical disease—for the mouth and throat, eye, ear, nose, vagina, rectum, urethra.—Probes, sounds, &c., Bougies and catheters.—Exploring and acupuncture needles.—Chemical tests, use of.—Effects of remedies.

The diseases are then taken up in alphabetical order, and the Diagnosis is made on the following system—

Taking, for example, the first subject treated.

Abscess—(abscedere, to separate) a circumscribed collection of pus (as contradistinguished from purulent infiltrations). Divided into (1) "acute," "phlegmonous," "hot;" and (2) "chronic" or "cold," according to the presence or not of acute inflammatory action. The description is then given of the signs and symptoms of Acute Abscess, followed by a description of other diseases that may be confounded with it (local œdema of the cellular tissue in the neighborhood of joints, and Aneurism), showing wherein they differ.

The author then describes Cold or Chronic Abscess, showing how Lipoma Cysts and Hydated Tumours, Hernia, Soft Cancer, and Aneurism, are sometimes confounded with it, and the symptoms wherein they differ.

In the same manner all the Surgical Diseases are fully described.

The book has been reprinted from the advance sheets purchased from the author, is got up in the best style, and from the great reputation of the writer, both as a Surgeon and as a fluent composer, cannot fail to find its appropriate place in the hands of the Civil and Military practitioner.

which are of the most importance to the military surgeon. This was deemed advisable, in order to render the volume as convenient and portable as possible. Within these limits the constant effort has been to embrace the greatest number of subjects, to arrange them in the best form for reference, and to give the largest amount of practical details, anatomical and operative.

As the value of such a work is much enhanced by engravings, care has been taken to illustrate every subject to the fullest extent. For this purpose works on operative surgery have been largely consulted, and such illustrations selected as were deemed most valuable. To avoid frequent repetitions, no mention is made in the text of the source from which they have been derived, and this occasion is taken to make proper acknowledgment. In the chapter on Minor Surgery, the illustrations are copied from English surgical treatises, Sédillot's *Traité de Med. Operat.*, and Jamain's *Manuel de Petit Chir.*; the illustrations of the Operations on Arteries are from Sédillot (*op. cit.*) and Guérin's *Elem. de Chir. Operat.*; in the chapter on Amputations, the illustrations are from English works, viz. Skey, Fergusson, Liston, Guthrie, and Druitt, and from Guérin (*op. cit.*), Chassaignac's *Traité Clinique et Pratique des Operations Chirurgicales, &c.*, and Bernard and Huette's *Illustrated Manual of Operative Surgery and Surgical Anatomy*; in the chapter on Resections, the illustrations of operations are from Chassaignac (*op. cit.*), Guthrie, Heyfelder's *Operationslehre und Statistic der Resectionen*, Erichsen, and Bernard and Huette (*op. cit.*). The illustrations of instruments through the volume have been selected by Tiemann & Co., and Wade & Ford, Instrument Makers of this city, and generally represent the latest improvements.

Although this work is limited, as stated above, yet the subjects treated are, with the exception of Gunshot Wounds, such as constantly engage the attention of the surgeon in civil and hospital practice, and it is believed that it will prove to this class of practitioners a useful and acceptable aid to the memory. To the students of Operative Surgery, it presents in sufficient detail for the purposes of study and practice, the methods of performing the ordinary operations in Surgery.

AMERICAN MEDICAL TIMES.—Complete sets of this valuable Journal can be had in half yearly Vols., in cloth or in numbers. Vol. I. 4to. (July to December, 1860), to Vol. VIII. (January to June, 1864). Price $2.00 per Vol. in cloth, or $1.50 per Vol. in numbers.

BAUDENS.—On Military and Camp Hospitals, and the Health of Troops in the Field. Being the results of a Commission to inspect the Sanitary Arrangements of the French Army, and incidentally of other Armies in the Crimean War. 12mo. New York, 1862. $1.25.

BELL.—Knowledge of Living Things, with the Law of their Existence. 12mo., with 2 Colored Plates and 60 Woodcuts. New York. $1.

BERNARD & HUETTE.—Illustrated Manual of Operative Surgery and Surgical Anatomy. Edited, with Notes and Additions, by W. H. Van Buren, M.D., Professor of Anatomy, University Medical College, and C. E. Isaacs, M.D. Complete in one Volume, 8vo., with 113 Colored Plates, half-bound Morocco, gilt tops. 1856. $30.00.

BLAKE.—Report of a Geological Reconnoissance in California, made in Connexion with the Expedition to Survey Routes in California, under Lieut. Williamson, with an Appendix by Profs. Agassiz, Gould, Bailey, Conrad, Torrey, Schæffer, and Easton. Profusely and magnificently Illustrated. 4to. New York, 1858. Cloth. $8.00.

BLOWPIPE.—A System of Instruction in the Practical Use of the Blowpipe, being a Graduated Course of Analysis for the use of Students and all those engaged in the Examination of Metallic Combinations. 12mo. 269 pages, fully Illustrated. New York, 1858. $1.50.

CHAVASSE.—Advice to a Mother on the Management of her Offspring. 12mo. 50 cts.

EDWARDS (A. M.).—Life Beneath the Waters; or, the Aquarium in America. Illustrated by Plates and Woodcuts drawn from Life. 12mo. New York. $1.50.

GESNER (A.).—A Practical Treatise on Coal, Petroleum, and other Distilled Oils. 8vo., fully Illustrated. New York. $1.50.
"The most complete and practical work on the subject."

ISHERWOOD (B. T.), Engineer-in-Chief, U.S.N. Engineering Precedents for Steam Machinery, embracing the Performances of Steamships, Experiments with Propelling Instruments, Condensers, Boilers, etc.; accompanied by Analyses of the same: the whole being original matter, and arranged in the most practical and useful manner for Engineers. Vol. 1, 8vo. Illustrated. New York. 1859. $1.25.
——— Vol. 2, 8vo. Illustrated. New York, 1859. $2.50.

JACOBI.—Dentition and its Derangements. A Course of Lectures delivered in the New York Medical College. 12mo. New York, 1862. $1.25.

MOREL.—Elements of Human Histology, Translated and Adapted to the Wants of the American Students. By W. H. Van Buren. 1 Vol., 8vo. 28 Plates. Cloth, $3.00

OTTO.—Manual of the Detection of Poisons by Medico-Chemical Analysis. By J. Otto, Professor of Chemistry in Brunswick, Germany. Edited with Notes by W. Elderhorst. With Illustrations. 12mo. New York, 1857. $1.25.

RAFINESQUE (C. S.).—The Complete Writings of, on Recent and Fossil Conchology. Edited by W. G. Binney and G. W. Tryon, Jr. 8vo. New York. Illustrated. $2.50.

SAY (T.).—The Complete Writings of, on the Conchology of the United States. Edited by W. G. Binney.

This work consists of 252 pages of text, and 75 plates, containing 323 figures. It includes all the descriptions of genera and species ever published by Mr. Say, and also all his figures. It will therefore be the first and only complete edition of Say's Conchological Writings ever published, and the most extensive work on the general Conchology of the United States, since the greater number of known American species of mollusca were described by him.

The work also contains a very full index to all the generic and specific descriptions of Mr. Say, and to the synonyms used in his writings, with the name, date, volume, page, plate, and figure of the original works containing them.

Price of the work, bound in half-calf, with plain plates, 8vo. New York, 1858. $6.00.

Colored, $12.00.

It is hoped that the work will be encouraged not only by the conchologist, but also by all those desirous of placing the scattered and generally inaccessible writinge of the first and greatest American naturalist in a position to afford that assistance to science which their merit enables them to do.

——— The Complete Writings of, on the Entomology of North America. Edited by J. L. Le Conte, M.D., Member of the Academy of Natural Sciences of Philadelphia.

This work consists of 2 vols., 8vo., of 1226 pages and 55 plates, containing about 175 figures. Having purchased the original copper plates of the American Entomology, the drawings of which are so universally admired, and the plates being colored from specimens in the possession of Dr. Le Conte (not copied from the old plates), it is believed that nothing is wanting in the illustrations to render them worthy of the praise of Naturalists.

The work also contains a very full index to all the generic and specific descriptions of Mr. Say, and to the synonyms used in his writings, with the name, date, volume, page, plate, and figure of the original works containing them. Price of the work, 2 vols., 8vo. Colored plates, half-bound, red calf. New York, 1859. $20.00.

SMITH (Dr. S.).—Handbook of Surgical Operations. Fifth edition, Illustrated with 257 Engravings, 274 pages, 12mo., limp cloth. New York, 1863. $1.75.

*** The best and most complete work on the kind published.

SUCKLEY (G.), and COOPER (J. G.).—The Natural History of Washington Territory and Oregon, with much relating to Minnesota, Nebraska, Kansas, Utah, and California, between the thirty-sixth and forty-ninth parallels of Latitude. 4to., 58 Colored Plates. New York, 1860. $10.00.

TRYON (G. W., Jr.)—Academy Natural Science, Philadelphia. List of American Writers on Recent Conchology; with the Titles of their Memoirs, and Dates of Publication. January 1, 1861. 8vo.

Heavy plate paper, stitched, $1.00.

" " " cloth, $1.25.

VAN BUREN (W. H.).—See Bernard & Huette.

See Morel.

MITCHELL (J.).—Manual of Practical Assaying. For the Use of Metallurgists, Captains of Mines, and Assayers in General. Second Edition, much enlarged, with Illustrations, etc. 8vo. £1 1s.

CHEMICAL SOCIETY (Quarterly Journal of the). 15 vols. 8vo. London, 1848–62. Vols. 1 to 7 have been reduced to 8s. each. Vols. 8 to 15, 13s. each. Or in Quarterly Parts, price 3s. each. *The year* 1863 *is published Monthly at* 1*s. each.*

GRAHAM.—Elements of Chemistry; including the Application of the Science in the Arts. By T. Graham, F,R.S., L. and E., Master of the Mint, late Professor of Chemistry at University College, London. 2d Edition, revised and enlarged, copiously Illustrated with Woodcuts. 2 vols. 8vo 1850–1857. £2.

BOUSSINGAULT.—Rural Economy in its relation with Chemistry, Physics, and Meteorology. 8vo. 2d Edition, 18s.

CAMPBELL.—A Practical Text-Book of Inorganic Chemistry. 12mo 6s. 6d.

CHAPMAN.—Practical Mineralogy, 8vo., with 13 engravings. 7s.

———— Brief Descriptions of the Characters of Minerals. 12mo. Fig. 4s.

LIEBIG.—Chemistry and Physics. 8vo. 3s.

REID.—Rudiments of Chemistry. 12mo. Fig. 2s. 6d.

REGNAULT.—Elementary Treatise on Crystallography. 8vo. Illustrated by 108 Woodcuts. 3s.

THOMSON.—Chemistry of Organic Bodies: Vegetables. 8vo. £1 4s.

———— Heat and Electricity, 2d edition. 8vo. 15s.

KÆMPTS.—A Complete Course of Meteorology. By L. F. Kæmptz, Professor of Physics at the University of Halle. With Notes by Ch. Martins, and an Appendix by L. Lalanne. Translated, with Additions, by C. V. Walker. 1 vol., post 8vo., pp. 624, with 15 Plates, cloth boards. 1845. 12s. 6d.

MOQUIN-TANDON.—Manual of Medical Zoology: being a Detailed Description of Animals useful in Medicine, and the species hurtful to Man; with General Considerations on the Organization and Classification of Animals, and with a Resumé of the Natural History of Man. Edited, with Notes and Additions, by T Hulme, Esq. With 124 Wood Engravings, post 8vo. 1861. 12s. 6d.

QUEKETT (J.).—Lectures on Histology, delivered at the Royal College of Surgeons of England, containing Elementary Tissues of Plants and Animals, the Structure of the Skeletons of Plants and Vertebrate Animals. 2 vols. Illustrated by 340 Woodcuts. London, 1852–1854. £1 8s. 6d.

QUEKETT (J.).—Practical Treatise on the Use of the Microscope. Illustrated with 11 Steel Plates and 300 Wood Engravings. 8vo. 3d edition. London, 1855. £1 1s.

WEISBACH.—Mechanics of Machinery and Engineering. 2 vols. 8vo. With 900 Woodcuts. £1 19s.

NICHOL.—Architecture of the Heavens. Ninth Edition, 8vo., with 23 Steel Plates and many Woodcuts 1851. 16s.

FAU.—The Anatomy of the External Form of Man, for Artists, Painters, and Sculptors Edited by R. Knox, M.D., with Additions. 8vo. text, and 28 4to. Plates. London, 1849. Plain, £1 4s. Colored Plates, £2 2s.

NORMAN
PUBLISHING ®

Collaborators on the production of *The Army Surgeon's Manual*:

Jill Lustig, Project Manager
Seventeenth Street Studios, Designer
Martha Nicholson Steele, Editor
Technical Publications, Electronic Page Composition
Thomson-Shore, Printer and Binder

The display and text type for the new Introduction is Bodoni, a Postscript font from Adobe Systems.

This edition is limited to 750 copies.